SO-ABO-834

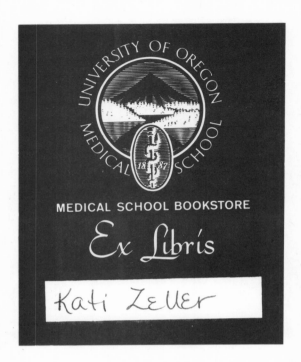

UNIVERSITY OF OREGON MEDICAL SCHOOL

18 87

MEDICAL SCHOOL BOOKSTORE

Ex Libris

MEDICAL

TERMINOLOGY

MADE EASY

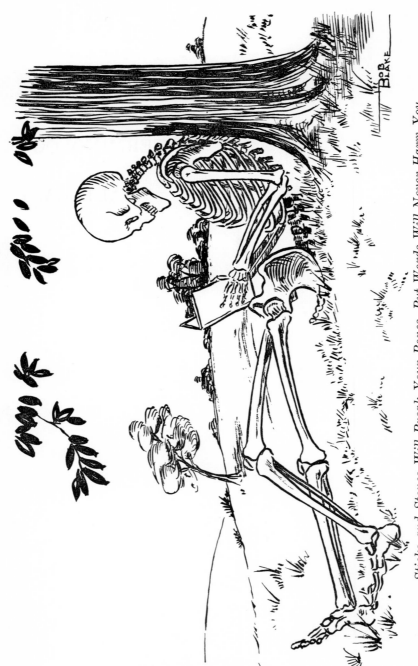

Sticks and Stones Will Break Your Bones, But Words Will Never Harm You.

MEDICAL TERMINOLOGY
MADE EASY

b y

JeHarned

Associate Professor, Emeritus
Duke University, Durham, North Carolina

SECOND EDITION

1968
Physicians' Record Company
Berwyn, Illinois

Library of Congress Catalog Card Number: 68-24088

Printed in the United States of America by the
Press of Physicians' Record Company, Berwyn, Illinois.

To the memory

of

DR. MALCOLM T. MACEACHERN

who in his long tenure with the American College
of Surgeons and American Hospital Association
encouraged, beyond measure, all medical and paramedical persons, in a trend toward betterment of
health to mankind

FOREWORD

MEDICAL practice, medical education, and hospitals cannot function without medical records, and medical records are useless without a uniform medical terminology, which all of the profession understand. This book, MEDICAL TERMINOLOGY MADE EASY, more than lives up to its name. Everyone of us in medicine and nursing and administration needs the instruction contained in this book.

For the student beginning preparation for medicine and other health careers, the introduction to the origin of medical words will be of great assistance. Most students of this generation have not had a background in Latin and Greek so that they can decipher the origin of medical words, but they can rely on this book to provide meaningful background. Medicine has grown up over many centuries and there are contributions from every language, Hebrew, Greek, Latin, French and English, which form our present medical terminology. It is interesting that in old languages, such as Chinese, which lacks many of the modern medical terms, the English word is inserted in toto because it cannot be translated into ideograms. Here again this book is useful to foreign students.

To most of us who rely upon abbreviations and symbols, this book is indispensable because it contains those abbreviations which are agreed upon by all English-speaking people. No less useful is the comprehensive indexing and the section correlating medical terminology with common lay terms for disease, symptoms and body structure.

In fact, each chapter shows in a basic way how this ordinarily incomprehensible language grows to comprehension for those training and working in premedical and paramedical fields.

W. C. DAVISON, M.D.
James B. Duke Professor of Pediatrics
and
Dean of Duke University School of
Medicine (1927-1960), Emeritus
Durham, North Carolina

FOREWORD TO THE FIRST EDITION

THE art and science of keeping medical records has come a long way since the turn of the century. Then medical records were poor in quality and, in fact, nonexistent in most hospitals. Indeed, it may be claimed that the evolution of systematic medical record keeping dates from the beginning of Hospital Standardization, and the progress has been steady and substantial.

The author of this book has bravely stepped into a new area of dissertation which is most timely. More complete development of the training of medical record librarians and of procedures to insure the accuracy of filing and cross-indexing of diseases and operations in the hospital are herein discussed. She has developed this work out of a vast practical experience and knowledge of medical terminology as well as from extensive research on this and related subjects.

There is much need for a basic, accurate and comprehensive terminology beyond that needed in the education and training of medical record librarians and development of disease indices. There is its value in research, in medical literature, and in statistical studies. Such a work assures greater accuracy and uniformity in recording diagnoses and end results.

From this textbook many will benefit — students, physicians, health workers, vital statistical and medical service workers of all kinds. It is a contribution that marks another important step in the advance of medical record keeping.

MALCOLM T. MACEACHERN, M.D.
Director Emeritus
American College of Surgeons
and
Professor and Director
Program in Hospital Administration
Northwestern University

PREFACE

THIS book will not teach the reader any medicine, even if he or she is misguided enough to learn every page by heart. It is not intended to do so. Specifically, its aim is to introduce beginners in the broadening field of medical work to the language of physicians. It is more than a phrasebook, but nothing like a grammar. It does not claim for its contents any etymological merits greater than those of the authorities consulted; arguments as to the use of words can always occur. It is certainly not a substitute for a medical dictionary. It offers to the medically uninitiated some practical help in understanding the polyglot (derived from Latin and Greek) vocabulary of physicians and surgeons. It is, in short, a special presentation on the current usages of words, culled from existing sources and my own experience.

If any justification for a special presentation is needed, it may be found in the truism that orderly study of any subject is preferable to haphazard study. It follows that orderly study should be arranged to meet the needs of the particular student. I hope this book may be useful to many people, including administrators of hospitals, premedical and first-year medical students, nurses, psychologists, medical record librarians, medical librarians, medical social workers, dietitians, physical therapists, hospital laboratory technicians, hospital x-ray technicians, medical secretaries, medical insurance adjustors and others. It is intended for the new recruit to the medical world — the novice in this field who has chosen some one of the many hospital or medical careers which offers a longed-for opportunity to hew wood and draw water for Aesculapius,[1] and who, in the very first week, is dismayed by the discovery that for every word the Greeks had, the Romans had another.

Durham, N. C. JeHarned

---

[1] Aesculapius: Greek god of healing.

ACKNOWLEDGEMENTS

IN THE preparation of even the most modest work dealing with medical words and their meanings, one must draw from many sources. For this book I have consulted several medical dictionaries and works on the origins and derivations of medical words, and many other books; and I have sought information and guidance from many people. I have referred to Dorland's *American Illustrated Medical Dictionary* and *Gould's Medical Dictionary*. Other books which I have consulted are: *The Origin of Medical Terms* by Henry Alan Skinner, M.B., F.R.C.S. (C); *Medical Greek and Latin at a Glance* by Walter R. Agard, B.Litt. (Oxon); *Medical Etymology* by O. H. Perry Pepper, M.D.; *The Language of Medicine* by R. F. Campbell, A.M., M.D.; *Medical Greek* by Achilles Rose; *Medical Records in the Hospital* by Malcolm T. MacEachern, M.D., C.M., D.Sc.; *The Standard Nomenclature of Diseases and Operations* published by American Medical Association; and *The Directory of Medical Specialists*. I am also indebted to Walter Winchell for permitting quotes from his column.

I greatly appreciate the help given by medical friends at Duke University Medical Center, whose ever ready assistance inspired me in ways too numerous to recount.

JeHARNED

Durham, N. C.

CONTENTS

CHAPTER I

CHAPTER II

  1. Meanings
  2. Spelling
  3. Pronunciation

CHAPTER III

  (A list and explanation of commonly recognized
  practices in medicine.)

CHAPTER IV

  1. Indicating location and direction
  2. Indicating negation
  3. Indicating number and measurement
  4. Indicating color
  5. Indicating position
  6. Miscellaneous

CHAPTER V

Part I

  1. Denoting relation and condition
  2. Miscellaneous suffixes

Part II

  1. Suffixes, words and phrases on operative terminology

CHAPTER VI

CHAPTER VII

CHAPTER VIII

CHAPTER IX

CHAPTER X

LIST OF ILLUSTRATIONS

CHAPTER I

INTRODUCTION TO THE ORIGIN OF
MEDICAL WORDS

EVERY PROFESSION, every trade, has its jargon, incomprehensible to the uninitiated. To a sailor, a rope is something to bend, hitch or reeve, never something to tie knots in. *Nolo contendere,*[1] estop,[2] *nolle prosequi,*[3] *nunc pro tunc,*[4] and torts are among the lawyer's verbal small change. The engineer's foot-pounds have neither length nor weight. The surveyor's chain has nothing to do with his watch. The very rogues have a diction which is to them incomparably more precise than the most eloquent English. Does not "snatch" (for kidnapping), for instance, not merely name the crime, but describe it too? *However, professional jargon, mysterious as it may sound to outsiders, is, for the purposes of each particular calling, more precise and less liable to errors of interpretation than ordinary English.* Commonly, a jargon word is coined specifically to name or describe a thing or act existing or done in a particular circumstance. A thing or act which is only similar (not identical) in itself and its circumstances is not entitled to the jargon name or description. New practitioners of every profession soon find that its jargon vocabulary expresses their professional thoughts and deeds with an accuracy and unmistakableness which they cannot attain by any other language.

---

[1] *Nolo contendere* — The name of a plea in a criminal action having the same legal effect as a plea of guilty, so far as regards all proceedings on the indictment, and on which the defendant may be sentenced. Commonly used to indicate no contest on the part of the defendant.

[2] Estop — To stop, bar or impede; to prevent; to preclude.

[3] *Nolle prosequi* — A formal entry in a civil or criminal action in which the plaintiff or prosecution declares he will not further prosecute the case.

[4] *Nunc pro tunc* — Now for then. A phrase applied to acts allowed to be done after the time when they should be done, with a retroactive effect.

Ref.: HENRY K. BLACK, *Black's Law Dictionary* (Third edition; St. Paul: West Publishing Co.).

So it is with medical jargon. Should there be any who think that to call medical terminology jargon is impolite to the medical profession, let it be mentioned that in *Webster's New International Dictionary* (Second Edition) jargon is defined as "a *hybrid* speech arising from a mixture of languages." Medical terminology is a hybrid speech. Physicians can, with the aid of their special vocabulary, name and describe the things they see and the things they do, more clearly and more precisely than anyone employing only the terms of common English usage. It is not that there is deeper merit in a medical term than in a nonmedical term having the same general meaning. *Talipes,* for instance (*talus,* ankle; *pes,* foot), is not as expressive a term as *clubfoot.* But the medical term is found to convey a shade of meaning not present in the nonmedical term. *Clubfoot* does not distinguish between all the types such as *talipes arcuatus, talipes calcaneus, talipes cavus, talipes equinus, talipes percavus, talipes planus, talipes valgus, talipes varus:* not to mention the combinations *equinovalgus, equinovarus, calcaneovalgus, calcaneovarus* and others. Nor could *clubfoot* be qualified to distinguish these varieties of *talipes* without using whole descriptive phrases, e.g., *resembling the hoof of a horse* for *equinovarus.* The plain fact is that the jargon has, over the years, acquired a precision of meaning which in many cases cannot be expressed in ordinary speech without comparative verbosity.

Two facts about medical terminology should be firmly lodged in the student's memory:

(1) Although largely modeled on classical (i.e., "dead") tongues, drawing freely, and at times recklessly, on Greek and Latin stems, prefixes and suffixes, medical terminology is as much a living and growing language as English itself. Hundreds of new words are born into it and hundreds die of disuse in each medical generation.

(2) Medical terminology grows, not by rules, but by the decisions of those who use it. Failing to find a word to describe some new thing or new act, the physician makes no bones about constructing a word which satisfies him.

Look in your medical dictionary for *melanoptysis* and you will not find it, but in the next edition it may be there. An English physician in 1947, wishing to record all instances of "black spit" among coalminers, used the word. Undismayed by the discovery that it did not appear in any of the medical dictionaries then consulted, this physician refused to give it up.

The dominance of Greek and Latin as source languages for physicians need not distress the student. But it would be foolish to deny the immense value of an educational background including these languages. Perry Pepper[1] deplores the fact that Latin and Greek are nowadays closed books to ninety-nine out of every hundred students, and he is right to do so. Yet, fortunately, prior acquaintance with them is not indispensable to the student who would learn medical terms. A knowledge of the components and the modes of construction of medical terms can be acquired with reasonable effort. The interested student will find himself familiar with many of the Latin and Greek roots and prefixes without effort. This knowledge will, of itself, encourage and stimulate the curious mind to obtain more. When this happens, a moderate facility in reading, writing and speaking the new language will not be long delayed. This is said confidently since the study of medical terminology has often fascinated beginners who refused to be intimidated.

Medical words are not monotonous; each separate syllable holds a meaning. That the modern meaning is frequently quite at variance with the original meaning only adds to the fascination. An idiot, according to the medical dictionary of today, is "a person without intellect and understanding; a feeble-minded person whose mental age is below two years." The Greek word *idiotes,* parent of the modern term, meant "private citizen": a man who held no public office. In such a civic-minded community, small wonder that those who never held office were looked upon as being of inferior mental capacity. *Idiot* therefore came to mean not a private citizen, but one ignorant of and incapable of taking

[1]O. H. Perry Pepper, M.D., *Medical Etymology* (Philadelphia, Pa.: W. B. Saunders Company).

part in public affairs. This was but a short step to the modern definition.

The fact that medical terminology owes so much to ancient tongues should not cause the student to expect purity in the beginning of any medical terms. The men who, down the ages, have coined new terms may have been good doctors, but they have not always been good philologists or good linguists. A mixture of roots from both languages, or a Greek prefix to a Latin stem, perhaps with a Greek suffix to finish off, seems to offend no medical ear. Words such as these are called *hybrids*. Here are a few examples:

EPILEPTIFORM	(Gr. *epileptos*, L. *forma*)
ENDOCERVICITIS	(Gr. *endon*, L. *cervix*, Gr. *itis*)
EXTRASYSTOLE	(L. *extra*, Gr. *systole*)
GRANULOCYTOPENIA	(L. *granulum*, Gr. *kytos*, Gr. *penia*)
SUBSTERNAL	(L. *sub*, Gr. *sternon*)

Indeed, the physicians are sometimes systematically, if barbarously, bilingual, since most anatomical terms are Latin, while inflammations of the parts are named in Greek.

Examples:

PART	LATIN	GREEK	DISEASE
Skin	*Cutis*	*Derma*	Dermatitis
Gland	*Glandula*	*Aden*	Adenitis
Breast	*Mamma*	*Mastos*	Mastitis
Marrow	*Medulla*	*Myelos*	Myelitis
Muscle	*Musculus*	*Mys*	Myositis
Kidney	*Ren*	*Nephros*	Nephritis
Stomach	*Stomachus*	*Gaster*	Gastritis
Womb	*Uterus*	*Metra*	Metritis

Lest it be thought the physician is the only or even the chief offender against etymological propriety, it is but just to say that by comparison with the modern journalist the medico is a literary purist. *Arteria* was originally the Greek word for air duct; Harvey filled it with blood and added *artery* to the physician's wordbook; the newspaperman has now driven his automobile into it and created the *arterial road* or, in his more colorful phrasing, the *traffic artery*. But none need be astonished by any philological crime committed by a profession which can write of "breaking down bottlenecks." It is not so long ago that a nationally known columnist (Walter Winchell) wrote that a certain racehorse had won several "consekkutif" races. Who knows but that this gem of jocularity may one day grace a dictionary? For out of the mass of "jitterbug" verbiage invented by each generation, some words always survive and pass into the language.

Hospitals and clinics, too, had humble beginnings. When the population of the world was small, travel hazardous and few men were skilled in medicine, families carried their sick to a crossroads, there to await some passerby who might recognize the malady and suggest a remedy. The aggregation of several such families was the precursor of the modern outpatient clinic. The beginnings of modern medical terminology were doubtless as casual — wrong meanings, false analogies, corruptions, exaggerations, scraps of half-remembered learning — all these have combined to produce a jargon which, down the years, has become a language.

To illustrate how, in the course of time, medical terms are altered, let us look at one of the most familiar word-endings in medicine, viz., *itis*, meaning an inflammatory condition. In an earlier era the term was *nosositis*, the word *nosos* meaning disease. Adding *nosositis* to an already cumbersome word denoting an anatomical part sometimes produced a difficult mouthful, so *nosos* was sacrificed. Today, for *appendinosositis* we have *appendicitis*, and for *cholecystonosositis* we have *cholecystitis*. We should be grateful, for the modern terms are not merely shorter, they are also more euphonious. The shortening process is active today; sometimes a word is shortened by a syllable, sometimes by a letter. An American physician, when he removes a patient's appendix, performs an *appendectomy;* his English colleague, doing the same thing, performs an *appendicectomy*. An American medical dictionary lists *etiology, anesthetic, orthopedic, hemorrhage;* an English lexicon will give *aetiology, anaesthetic, orthopaedic, haemorrhage*. *Melancholia* was the ancient physician's name for a condition which he believed to arise from black bile in the patient; today it is a term employed more by poets than physicians. *Brachium* meant arm; in the modern dictionary it now means *brace*. In medical language the original meaning survives in *brachial*. Physicians for centuries have appropriated words, altered them, discarded them and misused them, and, as a result, now have almost a special language in which they can communicate with each other.

The task of the newcomer is to learn this language within a reasonable time. The risk of "putting one's foot in it" may loom like a spectre over every faltering utterance until the medical jargon has been learned.

The *plan of study* recommended is simple. It includes *only* analysis of the basic structure of medical words, memorizing some of the commonest components, the study of examples, and some labor at exercises. The analytical phase is particularly interesting. Think of the word *pilonidal*, from *pilus* (hair) and *nidus* (nest), meaning literally, a nest of hairs. To the physician, a *pilonidal cyst* is a cavity containing hair. It is something which becomes infected and must be removed. But the normally curious will wonder why such cavities exist, and curiosity will not be lessened by the discovery that pilonidal cysts are usually located in the hinder part of the sufferer. The anthropologist may say learnedly that a pilonidal cyst is a retrocession and perhaps may believe that the pilonidal cyst is a hand-me-down from ape ancestry, concealed in this cystic manner by nature itself. The fledgling in medical terminology will get more fun out of connecting it with the John T. Scopes trial on evolution in Dayton, Tennessee, and William Jennings Bryan's part in the prosecution, as well as the much-quoted saying of Bryan: "I do not believe we have descended from monkeys, but am certain we are going to the dogs." In studying medical terminology, or any subject for that matter, it is much more easily learned if we connect our mental functioning with some such narrative or theorize practically for a moment on the origin of our subject.

CHAPTER II

PREREQUISITES TO MASTERY OF
MEDICAL TERMINOLOGY

MEDICAL TERMINOLOGY exists only for the purposes of medicine. Its purpose is to describe the human body, its functions, its normal state, its abnormal states, the diseases and injuries which affect it, and the various means, agents and procedures employed to prevent, minimize or cure the effects of disease and injury. Medical vocabulary is extensive, and many words in it are deceptively like other words. Complete familiarity with it is the only insurance against errors in interpretation and use.

Complete familiarity can be obtained only if the student knows: (a) *the precise meaning of each word,* (b) *the exact spelling of each word,* (c) *the correct pronunciation of each word.*

MEANINGS

The meanings of medical words are discoverable by analysis of the words themselves. Each word contains one or more *roots* or *stems.* To stems are affixed, fore or aft, *prefixes* and *suffixes.* The function of these affixed parts is to *add* information which helps in interpretation. It describes them more fully and locates them more precisely. It states how, when or why (or how, when *and* why) things were done to them.

Example:

Prefix	*Stem*	*Suffix*	*Medical Word*
ENDO-	CARD	-ITIS	ENDOCARDITIS
(within)	(heart)	(inflammation)	(Inflammation of the lining of the heart: the endocardium)

[7]

There is no limit to the number of stems which may be compounded together in a medical word, nor the number of prefixes or suffixes which may be employed in combination with them. The test of a good medical word is its descriptive aptness. However, in order to correctly form a word consisting of parts compounded, one must take note of the proper use of connective vowels. Vowels most commonly used are *o, i,* and sometimes *u.*

Example: neur(o)logy; germ(i)cidal; gran(u)lation.

It is possible to "pick up" medical word stems over a long period of association with physicians, but a more rapid acquaintance with them may be obtained by committing to memory some which are most frequently encountered. The same procedure will be found satisfactory with both prefixes and suffixes.

Care must be taken to make sure that the meanings of the stems, prefixes and suffixes are fully understood. The misinterpretation or omission of a single letter may completely alter a meaning — even reverse it — with, conceivably, actual harm to a patient, and, assuredly, a disastrous effect on one's standing with the medical profession.

SPELLING

In the process of analyzing medical words by breaking them down into meaningful parts, no pains must be spared to acquire accuracy in spelling. Misspelling in any language is a bad habit. It gives the impression of carelessness and inattention. It is fashionable (among bad spellers) to decry insistence on perfect spelling as an affectation of being learned, but this is easily countered. The feeling that bad spelling is the mark of the quick thinker is as ill-founded. So far as medical personnel is concerned, the unalterable truth is that misspelling a word may easily change its meaning. Again the sufferer *may* be the patient, and most certainly the sufferer *will* be the individual who commits the crime of misspelling.

PRONUNCIATION

Another kind of care is needed for the acquisition of good pronunciation. In learning any language, the student finds it hard to reach the point of utterance. He is especially diffident in the presence of others, particularly if the other person is fluent in the tongue he is attempting to learn. There are two aids to pronunciation available. The first is the pronouncing dictionary, in which the values and accents are designated by symbols. The second, and more important, is the student's own ear. Listen to physicians, mark how they pronounce medical words. Then try them over in private. Try them on lay friends who will not recognize mistakes. As confidence comes, take the plunge. Speak the words to those who know them. Do not back away at this stage. Do not mumble or slur the words. Come out with them, clear and distinct, and, at the next opportunity, the inhibition will have vanished. Misspelling and mispronunciation go together; habitual carelessness in pronunciation makes misspelling virtually certain.

Pitfalls are far from rare. Some stems, prefixes and suffixes have similarities of sound and only slight difference in spelling, like the words *too, to* and *two,* which are now taught to first graders as homonyms. They can easily be confused and require extra care in learning.

Examples in Medicine:

Word or Prefix	*Meaning*
My	Muscle
Py	Pus
Oral	Mouth
Aural	Ear
Urology	to do with urine and urinary tract
Neurology	to do with nervous system
Pyel	Kidney pelvis
Myel	Marrow
Ileum	Part of small intestine
Ilium	One of the pelvic bones

There are, of course, words which may be acceptably pronounced in more than one way.

Examples:

NEURASTHENIA	Newra'stheenia — Newra'sthen'ia
OLECRANON	O-lek'ran-on — O-lek-ra'non
ABDOMEN	Abdo'men — Ab'domen

Some words are differently pronounced in different parts of the English-speaking world.

Examples:

LABORATORY	lab'oratory — labor'atory
CERVICAL	servicle — ser-vī'cal
GYNECOLOGY	jin-ecol'ogy — jine-cology — gine-cology
MIGRAINE	mig-rain — mee-graine — my'grain
-ITIS	ītis — ētis
ANESTHETIST	A-ness'thet-ist — A-neess'thet-ist

The student will wish to know how to navigate all these tricky shoals. The answer is twofold — use your ear, listen carefully to local usage, and use your tongue, do not hesitate to ask the physician for meanings, spellings and pronunciations. In reading, study every unfamiliar term in relation to the preceding and succeeding context, consult the dictionary freely, and make a note of all words about which any doubt remains in your mind. In conversing, do not let an unfamiliar word pass without asking the user to say it again, to spell it and to tell you its meaning. At the earliest opportunity, write the word, look it up and construct a sentence in which it occurs correctly. (Then don't ask *anyone* about *that* word a second time!)

Above all, when using medical terminology in conversation, vocalize clearly. Do not slur. If anything, be on the side of over-enunciation. By this means you will avoid confusion. Slipshod pronunciation is the sign of imperfect knowledge.

There is beauty of sound in medical words and it is not far to seek. What could be more euphonious than *syringomyelia?* This thought of euphony occurred to novelist Susan Ertz, who made Madame Claire[1] write to a sick friend:

---

[1] Susan Ertz, *Madame Claire* (New York: Appleton-Century-Crofts, Inc.).

"I am so sorry you are feeling less well. How is the phlebitis? No one ought to suffer from anything with such a pretty name. Did you ever stop to think that the names of diseases and the names of flowers are very similar? For instance, I might say, 'Do come and see my garden. It is at its best now, and the double pneumonias are really wonderful. I suppose the mild winter had something to do with that. I am very proud of my trailing phlebitis, too, and the laryngitises and the deep purple quinsies are a sight to behold. The bed of asthmas and malarias that you used to admire is finer than ever this summer, and the dear little dropsies down by the lake make such a pretty showing with the blue of the anthrax border behind them.' "

So look closely at your medical terms; take a second look. Concentrate upon the spelling. Roll them around in your oral fossae. Say them. Repeat them over again. Make them alive and worthy of their portent. Extol the simplicity of their growth. Bury your interest in and share their derivative romance. Live with them. Work over them. Learn them. Know the beauty of their sound and the oftentimes sordidness of their meaning. In other words, let none pass as just another word until you have reasonably mastered it.

CHAPTER III

GENERAL AND SPECIAL PRACTICES
IN MEDICINE

THE FIRST plunge into the ocean of medical terminology is to make the acquaintance of the types of practice in which physicians are trained.

The practice of medicine and surgery may be divided into two broad categories, viz., *general* practice and *specialist* practice.

The general practitioner (nowadays usually known as the "L.M.D.," "Local M.D., the family physician or the physician at hand"), is normally the first resort of the sick person, and the specialist gives the second opinion. Ideally, the specialist is called in on the initiative of the family physician when the latter recognizes or suspects a condition in which advice from the appropriate specialist, as to diagnosis or treatment or both, will be valuable.

The larger or teaching hospitals usually employ staffs of whom the majority are specialists. In referring a patient to the hospital, the family physician often seeks specialist opinion as to diagnosis and treatment, but he may retain his privilege as ATTENDING PHYSICIAN. If his patient is turned over to another physician for complete care, the family physician becomes the REFERRING PHYSICIAN. At times a patient is sent to a hospital so that he may receive special ancillary or nursing care which is not available at home. In many instances, domestic and economic factors have a bearing on the medical treatment and hospitalization. In rural areas and small towns remote from greater medical facilities, the family physician will of necessity treat to a conclusion many patients who would, in other circumstances, be referred directly to specialists, in or out of a hospital.

Specialist practice is subdivided into:

(a) *clinical specialism,* in which the specialist limits his practice to the treatment of certain diseases or to the diseases of a single organ, or diseases occurring within a specific anatomical system of the body, or of a single class of patients, or the application of a single method of treatment, and

(b) *hospital departmental specialism,* in which the specialist devotes himself to the practice of certain techniques of examination, or to the administration and use of certain substances, agents or equipment, or to the teaching of students in one or more branches of medical knowledge.

A clinician (Gr. *klinê* = bed) is a physician (*physis* = nature; *ician* = one versed in) whose opinions, teachings and treatment are based upon experience at the bedside. A clinical specialist (or "service chief") is therefore one who personally sees, takes charge of, and directs the treatment of patients. A hospital departmental specialist, when acting in that capacity (e.g., the head of the pathology department), is not necessarily a clinician. Any diagnosis or direction of treatment by him is remote; i.e., it is not done on the ward, at the patient's bedside, or in the clinic.

Medical specialisms are made up of various practices in medicine and are divided into groups which are recognized by the *American Boards of Special Medical Practices.*[1] The American Boards are organized for improvement of standards of graduate medical education and training, and of the practice of medical specialties. These Boards evaluate and certify abilities in special medical practices.

The list of current American Medical Boards includes:

1. *Anesthesiology*
2. *Dermatology*
3. *Internal Medicine*

[1] *Directory of Medical Specialists,* Vol. X (Chicago: Marquis—Directory of Medical Specialists)

SUBSPECIALTIES

3.1 — *Allergy*
3.2 — *Cardiovascular Disease*
3.3 — *Gastroenterology*
3.4 — *Pulmonary Disease*

4. *Neurological Surgery*
5. *Obstetrics and Gynecology*
6. *Ophthalmology*
7. *Orthopedic Surgery*
8. *Otolaryngology*
9. *Pathology*
10. *Pediatrics*
11. *Physical Medicine and Rehabilitation*
12. *Plastic Surgery*
13. *Preventive Medicine*
14. *Proctology*
15. *Psychiatry and Neurology*
16. *Radiology*
17. *Surgery*
18. *Thoracic Surgery*
19. *Urology*

The *American Board of Anesthesiology* certifies the abilities of the Anesthesiologist.

ANESTHESIOLOGIST

A physician specializing in the study and practice of anesthesia. He may be in private or hospital practice or in the teaching field of anesthesia. This specialty covers the knowledge of anesthesia agents and the body reaction to their intake. It also includes the knowledge of technics of administration of anesthesia agents. The specialty is called ANESTHESIOLOGY.

(Note): Nurse-Anesthetist

The Nurse-Anesthetist is one fully qualified as a registered nurse who is specializing in administering anesthesia and does not fit in this classification of medical practices.

The *American Board of Dermatology and Syphilology* certifies the abilities of the Dermatologist and Syphilologist.

DERMATOLOGIST

A clinician specializing in the diagnosis and treatment of persons suffering from skin disorders. The specialty is called DERMATOLOGY. Sometimes this specialty is combined with Syphilology.

SYPHILOLOGIST

A clinician specializing in the diagnosis and treatment of syphilis (an infectious disease in which the infecting microorganism[1] is called *Treponema pallidum*). The specialty is called SYPHILOLOGY. Syphilology is usually associated with Public Health Services rather than with Hospital Medical Services.

The *American Board of Internal Medicine* certifies as to fundamental training and basic experience in this specialty and also certifies as to certain subspecialties which require the same medical background. These subspecialists are known as the Allergist, Cardiologist, Pulmonary Disease Specialist and Gastroenterologist.

INTERNIST

A clinician specializing in the diagnosis and nonsurgical treatment of adults suffering from internal diseases generally. The specialty is called INTERNAL MEDICINE.

SUBSPECIALISTS

ALLERGIST

A clinician specializing in the diagnosis and treatment of persons who have asthma, hay fever, certain types of skin

---

[1] Microorganism—any virus or bacterium which invades tissue and sets up an inflammatory process. "Micro" indicates that it is too small to be seen with the naked eye.

disease and those who are suspected of "sensitivity" reactions. The specialty is called ALLERGY.

CARDIOLOGIST

A clinician specializing in the diagnosis and treatment of persons suffering from disorders of the heart and vascular system. The specialty is called CARDIOLOGY.

GASTROENTEROLOGIST

A clinician specializing in the diagnosis and treatment of persons suffering from diseases of the stomach and intestines. The specialty is called GASTROENTEROLOGY.

PULMONARY DISEASE SPECIALIST

A clinician specializing in the diagnosis and treatment of persons suffering from diseases of the lungs, pleura, and mediastinal structures. The specialty is called PULMONARY DISEASES. A clinician who limits his practice to the diagnosis and treatment of tuberculosis of the lungs is called a PHTHISIOLOGIST (tiz-e-ol'o-jist). PHTHISIS is pulmonary (lung) tuberculosis.

The *American Board of Neurological Surgery* certifies the abilities of the Neurosurgeon.

NEUROSURGEON

A clinician specializing in the diagnosis and surgical treatment of persons suffering from diseases of the brain, spinal cord and peripheral nervous system. The specialty is called NEUROLOGICAL SURGERY.

The *American Board of Obstetrics and Gynecology* certifies the abilities of the Obstetrician and Gynecologist.

OBSTETRICIAN

A clinician specializing in the diagnosis and care of women during pregnancy, labor and the puerperium (the period of convalescence following labor). The specialty is called OBSTETRICS.

GYNECOLOGIST

A clinician specializing in the diagnosis and medical and surgical treatment of diseases of the female reproductive organs. The specialty is called GYNECOLOGY.

The *American Board of Ophthalmology* certifies the abilities of the Ophthalmologist.

OPHTHALMOLOGIST

A clinician specializing in the diagnosis, medical and surgical treatment of diseases of the eye, including visual defects correctable with glasses, muscle imbalances producing squints (cross-eyes) and other abnormalities of the ocular system. The specialty is called OPHTHALMOLOGY.

(Note): The ophthalmologist is not to be confused with either an optometrist or an optician. These are not medically trained practitioners, nor are they certified by any of the American Medical Boards. The optometrist is licensed in the State of his residence according to the laws of that State. His training and licensing allow him to examine vision and prescribe and provide lenses or visual training. He uses the initials O.D. An optician is a nonmedically trained practitioner who may grind, fit and supply eyeglasses.

The *American Board of Orthopedic Surgery* certifies the abilities of the Orthopedic Surgeon or Orthopedist.

ORTHOPEDIC SURGEON OR ORTHOPEDIST

A clinician specializing in the diagnosis and (mainly) surgical or manipulative treatment of bones, joints, and the system of locomotion. (Bones excluded are those of the head and anterior thorax.) The specialty is called ORTHOPEDICS.

The *American Board of Otolaryngology* certifies the abilities of the Otolaryngologist or Otorhinolaryngologist.

OTOLARYNGOLOGIST

A clinician specializing in the diagnosis and medical and surgical treatment of persons suffering from diseases of the ear, nose and throat (pharynx and larynx). The specialty is called OTORHINOLARYNGOLOGY or, shortened, OTOLARYNGOLOGY. Some specialists in this field limit their practice to the use of the *bronchoscope*. The art of applying this instrument is called *bronchoscopy* or *endoscopy*. The use of this instrument implies "looking into" or a "periscope view." The specialists themselves are called BRONCHOSCOPISTS or ENDOSCOPISTS.

The *American Board of Pathology* certifies the abilities of the Clinical Pathologist and Anatomical Pathologist. PATHOLOGY is the specialty in the practice of medicine dealing with the causes and nature of disease. It contributes to diagnosis and treatment through knowledge obtained by laboratory study of specimens from the body.

CLINICAL PATHOLOGIST

A medical specialist who is applying his special knowledge of pathology to the study of specimens dealing with bacteriology, biochemistry, immunology, parasitology, hematology, endocrinology, and clinical microscopy in relation to diagnosis, prognosis and treatment of clinical disease.

BACTERIOLOGY. The study of pathogenic (capable of causing disease) bacteria (microorganisms). In some hospitals, especially medical school hospitals, bacteriology is separated from pathology. In this case, the specialist is called the BACTERIOLOGIST.

BIOCHEMISTRY. The study of the chemistry of living organisms. A specialist in this field is the BIOCHEMIST, who is not invariably medically qualified. It is his duty to supervise technicians who carry out chemical tests necessary for diagnosis and treatment.

CYTOLOGY. The study of cells, their structures (differentiating normal and diseased cells) and their functions.

IMMUNOLOGY. The study of security against and resistance to disease.

PARASITOLOGY. The study of parasites and their hosts.

HEMATOLOGY. The study of the forms and structure of blood and blood-forming organs. Sometimes a specialist in internal medicine will limit his practices to diseases of the blood and blood-forming organs. If he does, his background must be the same as that of the Internist, and he is called a HEMATOLOGIST.

ENDOCRINOLOGY. The study of structures and functions of the glands of internal secretion in both male and female; i.e., the thyroid, parathyroid, ovarian, testes, adrenal, pancreatic, pituitary and pineal glands. If a physician limits his practice to diseases of these ductless glands, he is called an ENDOCRINOLOGIST.

CLINICAL MICROSCOPY. The study of the nature of disease, as it affects the structures and functions of the body, by use of the microscope.

ANATOMICAL PATHOLOGIST

A medical specialist who applies his knowledge of pathology to the description and diagnosis of gross and microscopic specimens. (Gross, or macroscopic, examination = examination by naked eye.)

The *American Board of Pediatrics* certifies the abilities of the Pediatrician.

PEDIATRICIAN

A clinician specializing in physical and mental child care, in both health and disease. The specialty is called PEDIATRICS. Note: Child age is generally considered to be from birth to between twelve and fourteen years of age, depending upon the development of the child. However, the current and coming trend seems to be that pediatric care should begin earlier than birth. Dr. Wilburt C. Davison, former Dean of the School of Medicine of Duke University and Professor of Pediatrics, states: "Pediatrics is child care in health and disease, both physical and mental, from *conception through adolescence.*" This unusual and perhaps controversial definition emphasizes that health of the child begins in the antenatal period through care of the mother, and also serves to emphasize the point that specialism in medicine cannot be rigidly defined because of overlapping of services.

The *American Board of Physical Medicine and Rehabilitation* certifies the abilities of the Physiatrist. The specialty may also be called PHYSIATRICS (fiz-e-at′riks).

PHYSIATRIST (fiz-e′at-rist)

A clinician specializing in the treatment of illnesses or defects which are remediable (wholly or partly) by the use of natural or physical agents, e.g., heat, light, air, water, electricity, exercise. Some of the diseases and conditions coming within this field are arthritis and the various types of rheumatism, neuromuscular and musculoskeletal diseases such as postpoliomyelitic deformities, cerebral palsy and paraplegia patients. A large group of post-traumatic and orthopedic conditions also fall into this category. REHABILITATION is included under this specialty due to the fact that many patients must be helped to return to useful life through the Physiatrist's guidance and encouragement. The patient is taught to rely on the able part of his mind and body mechanism. Therefore, it is also required that the Physiatrist have, as an integral part of this specialty, a knowledge of the role of associated personnel and the ability to coordinate their services. These associated personnel are Physical Therapists, Occupational Therapists, Clinical Psychologists, Social Service Workers and Vocational Counselors.

The *American Board of Plastic Surgery* certifies the abilities of the Plastic Surgeon.

PLASTIC SURGEON

A clinician specializing in surgical reconstruction of malformations of the body resulting from congenital, accidental or disease processes. The specialty is called PLASTIC SURGERY.

The *American Board of Preventive Medicine* certifies the abilities of Physicians who specialize in Public Health, in Occupational Medicine and in Aviation Medicine.

SPECIALIST IN PREVENTIVE MEDICINE

A clinician involved with the study, prevention and therapy of diseases with epidemiological significance. The specialty is called PREVENTIVE MEDICINE.

The *American Board of Proctology* certifies the abilities of the Proctologist.

PROCTOLOGIST

A clinician trained in the specialty which deals with the diagnosis and treatment of diseases and anomalies of the colon, the rectum and anal canal. The specialty is called PROCTOLOGY.

The *American Board of Psychiatry and Neurology* certifies the abilities of the Neurologist and the Neuropsychiatrist.

NEUROLOGIST

A clinician specializing in the diagnosis and treatment of persons suffering from diseases of the nervous system, especially the central nervous system. The specialty is called NEUROLOGY.

PSYCHIATRIST

A clinician specializing in the diagnosis and treatment of persons suffering from disorders of the mind. The specialty is called PSYCHIATRY or NEUROPSYCHIATRY.

The *American Board of Radiology* certifies the abilities of the Radiologist, Roentgenologist, Diagnostic Roentgenologist, and Therapeutic Radiologist.

RADIOLOGIST

A clinician who deals with the diagnosis and therapeutic application of radiant energy, including Roentgen[1] rays (deep X-ray therapy) and radium.

---

[1] Wilhelm Konrad Von Roentgen (Rent'gen), German physicist.

ROENTGENOLOGIST

A clinician in the specialty of radiology who deals with diagnostic and therapeutic application of Roentgen rays (X rays).

DIAGNOSTIC ROENTGENOLOGIST

A clinician in the specialty of radiology who deals exclusively in the study and use of X rays (or Roentgen rays) for the purpose of diagnosis.

THERAPEUTIC RADIOLOGIST

A clinician in the specialty of radiology who deals only in therapeutic application of Roentgen rays and radium.

The specialty of these preceding four categories is called RADIOLOGY.

The *American Board of Surgery* certifies the abilities of the General Surgeon and the Thoracic Surgeon.

GENERAL SURGEON

A clinician trained in the fundamental principles of the nature of injury and disease of the human body, and in their management by operative means. The specialty is called GENERAL SURGERY. Many physicians trained in the principles of general surgery have confined their practice to certain regions of the body (viz., Neurosurgeon, Thoracic Surgeon, Orthopedic Surgeon, Plastic Surgeon, etc.), and where General Surgeons work in group practice with these specialists, General Surgeons have relinquished that part of the practice of surgery to them. In many localities, however, General Surgeons continue the practice of surgery of the entire body, for their basic training has prepared them to take care of all except the very complicated diagnostic and operative procedures done in these other surgical specialty fields.

THORACIC SURGEON

A clinician specializing in the diagnosis and surgical treatment of persons suffering from diseases of the organs of the thorax (lungs, pleura, esophagus, mediastinal structures and heart). The specialty is called THORACIC SURGERY.

The *American Board of Surgical Urology* certifies the abilities of the Urologist.

UROLOGIST

A clinician specializing in the diagnosis and (mainly) surgical treatment of persons suffering from diseases of the urinary tract of the female and the genitourinary tract of the male. The specialty is called UROLOGY.

OTHER SPECIALISTS

DIABETIC SPECIALIST or DIABETICIAN

A clinician specializing in the diagnosis and treatment of persons suffering from diabetes mellitus. (Diabetes mellitus is a disease in which too much sugar is found in the blood stream. Sugar in the urine may or may not be found.) The specialty is usually called DIABETIC SPECIALTY. The Diabetic Specialist usually obtains his American Board certification under Internal Medicine.

GERIATRICIAN

A clinician specializing in the diagnosis and treatment of aged persons. The specialty is called GERIATRICS. The Geriatrician usually obtains his American Board certification under Internal Medicine.

DENTAL SURGEON or DENTIST and ORTHODONTIST

A clinician having a degree in dentistry (D.D.S. or D.M.D.) specializing in treatment of persons suffering from diseases of the teeth and in the prevention of dental disease. The specialty is called DENTAL SURGERY or DENTISTRY. The Orthodontist deals with the prevention and correction of irregularities of the teeth and malocclusion. These specialists obtain special affiliation with the American Dental Association.

ONCOLOGIST

A clinician specializing in the diagnosis and (mainly) surgical treatment of persons suffering from malignant neoplasms (cancer). The specialty is called ONCOLOGY.

ORAL SURGEON

A clinician specializing in the diagnosis and (mainly) surgical treatment of persons suffering from diseases of the mouth and its allied structures. The specialty is called ORAL SURGERY. The Oral Surgeon usually obtains his American Board certification under General Surgery and/or Plastic Surgery.

CLINICAL PSYCHOLOGIST

A psychologist trained in the special technics which are useful in clinics for Mental Hygiene and Child Guidance and in the psychiatric study of patients. The specialty is called CLINICAL PSYCHOLOGY.

SPECIALISTS IN TEACHING

EPIDEMIOLOGIST

One versed in diseases (especially communicable diseases) affecting large numbers of people. The specialty is called EPIDEMIOLOGY.

ANATOMIST

One (not invariably medically qualified) versed in the structure of the body and the relation of its parts. The specialty is called ANATOMY.

CLINICAL PHYSIOLOGIST

One versed in the study of the active functions of the body. The specialty is called CLINICAL PHYSIOLOGY.

PHARMACOLOGIST

One versed in the effects of drugs on the animal organism, especially the human body. The specialty is called PHARMACOLOGY.

The Prefixes and Their Stem

CHAPTER IV

PREFIXES[1] AND PSEUDO-PREFIXES

THE "TRUE PREFIX" is considered to be one or more letters or syllables combined at the beginning of a word to further explain or add to a meaning. For example, *un* as a forepart of a word expressing "not," "opposite," or "contrary to," is a prefix in many words. Examples are: uneven, unlawful, and unbecoming. But the forepart of every compound word is not necessarily a true prefix. Frequently the prefix is a noun or an adjective in its stem form. In the word "birthday," the so-called prefix is a noun; in "hardware" it is an adjective. Foreparts such as these may be called "pseudo-prefixes." They assume the character and use of the true prefix. Prefixes of either type may be used with the body or stem of many words to help express condition, location, size, direction, and many other qualities. An example of a true prefix in the medical vocabulary is *end,* meaning within. This prefix may be used with many stems indicating anatomical parts, as: *endocardium* (within the heart or heart lining), *endocranium* (within the skull — literally = a brain lining). Examples of pseudo-prefixes are found in words like *meningocele* (protrusion of brain lining), and *phlebectasia* (dilatation of a vein).

INSTRUCTION IN PREFIXES — The following lists will give many medical prefixes in both the true and pseudotypes. These lists consist only of the most commonly used terms. They may be learned best by rote; that is, by memory and re-use; by forming other words than the examples given of the prefix. Home assignments may be made by instructors in medical terminology by asking students to make lists of the prefixes, learn the meanings, and use them in other medical terms.

---

[1]Read: Walter R. Agard, *Medical Greek and Latin at a Glance* (New York: Paul B. Hoeber, Inc.).

Home work may be turned in each class period and corrected by the instructor. The instructor should remember the importance placed on pronunciation and spelling.

PREFIXES INDICATING LOCATION, DIRECTION, AND TENDENCY

Prefix	Meaning	Example
AB-	from, away from	**Abnormal,** away from normal
APO-		**Apoplexy,** a stroke from
DE-		**Deflect,** a bending from
AD-	to; near; toward	**Adrenal,** adjoining the kidney
AMBI-	both	**Ambidextrous,** able to use both hands equally well
AMPHI-	on both sides	**Amphicrania,** headache on both sides of the skull
AMPHO-		**Amphogenic,** producing offspring of both sexes
ANA-	up, apart, across	**Anabolism,** a building up
ANTE-	before	**Antepartum,** before delivery
PRE-		**Prenatal,** before birth
PRO-		**Prognosis,** a fore-knowing (forecast)
ANTI-	against	**Antiseptic,** an agent used against infection
CONTRA-		**Contraindicant** (kon-trah-in'dik-ant), indicating against
COUNTER-		**Counterirritant,** an agent which irritates, acting normally to combat some other condition

Prefix	*Meaning*	*Example*
CATA- KATA-	down	**Catabolism,** a throwing down or destructive reaction
CIRCUM-	around	**Circumocular,** around the eye
PERI-		**Pericardium,** membrane around the heart
CO-	with, together	**Coordination,** to work together
COM-		**Compound,** to mix or fuse together
CON-		**Congenital,** with birth
SYM-		**Symphysis** (sim′fis-is), a growing together
SYN-		**Synarthrosis,** a bony union
DIA-	through	**Diathermy,** a heating through
PER-		**Percussion,** a striking through
TRANS-		**Transurethral,** through the urethra
DI-	apart from	**Diarthrosis,** a joint apart (movable joint)
DIS-		**Disarticulation,** taking a joint apart
E-	out from	**Enucleate,** to shell out like a nut
EC-		**Eczema** (ek′ze-mah), to boil out from
EX-		**Exhale,** to breathe out
ECT-	outside	**Ectonuclear,** outside nucleus of cell

Prefix	Meaning	Example
EXO-	outside	**Exogenous** (ex-oj'en-us), produced outside
EXTRA-		**Extravasation,** outside its vessel
EM-	in	**Empyema,** pus inside a space, usually the pleural space
EN-		**Encapsulated,** in a capsule
IM-		**Impacted,** packed in
IN-		**Inspiration,** breathing in
END-	within	**Endometrium,** mucous membrane within the uterus
ENTO-		**Entocyte,** inner cell
INTRA-		**Intramuscular,** within the muscles
EPI-	upon	**Epicondyle,** an eminence upon a condyle
ESO-	inward	**Esotropia,** a turning inward of the eye (cross-eye)
INFRA-	under	**Infrapatellar,** under the kneecap
HYPO-		**Hypospadias** (hi-po-spa'de-as), urethra opens under the penis
SUB-		**Subclavian,** an artery running under the clavicle
INTER-	between	**Intercostal,** between the ribs
INTRO-	into	**Introflexion,** bending into or a leading into; inward

Prefix	*Meaning*	*Example*
META-	change	**Metaplasia,** a change in the character of a tissue
PARA-	beside	**Paravertebral,** beside the spine
POST-	after	**Postmortem,** after death
RE-	again	**Recurrence,** to occur again
RETRO-	backward	**Retroflexion,** a bending backward
RE-		**Relapse,** a slipping back
SUPER-	above	**Superciliary,** above area of eyebrow
SUPRA-		**Suprapubic,** above the pubic bone
ULTRA-	beyond or excess	**Ultrasterile,** excessively sterile

PREFIXES OF NEGATION

Prefix	*Meaning*	*Example*
A-	without	**Apnea,** without breathing
AN-		**Anesthetic,** without sensation
IM-	not	**Immature,** not mature
IN-		**Incurable,** not curable

PSEUDO-PREFIXES DENOTING NUMBER AND MEASUREMENT

Pseudo-Prefix	*Meaning*	*Example*
UNI-	one	**Unicellular,** consisting of one cell only
MON-		**Mononuclear,** a cell with a single nucleus

Pseudo-Prefix	*Meaning*	*Example*
BI-	two	**Bilateral,** affecting two sides
BIN-		**Binocular,** two-eyed
DI-		**Dicephalus** (di-sef'al-us), two heads
TER-	three	**Tertiary** (ter'she-a-re), the third stage
TRI-		**Tricellular,** three-celled
QUADR-	four	**Quadriceps femoris,** four combined muscles in the thigh
TETRA-		**Tetralogy of Fallot,** an anomaly of the heart, having four features
QUINQUE-	five	**Quinquecuspid** (kwin-kwe-kus'pid), a tooth having five points
PENT(A)-		**Pentachromic,** being able to distinguish only five colors
SEX-	six	**Sexdigitate,** having six fingers or toes
HEX(A)-		**Hexapod,** six-footed insect
SEPT-	seven	**Septipara** (sep-tip'ah-rah), a woman who has borne seven children
HEPTA-		**Heptad,** an element having power to combine with seven substances
OCTA-	eight	**Octagonal,** eight-sided
NONAGEN-	ninety	**Nonagenarian,** one who is ninety years old

Pseudo-Prefix	Meaning	Example
NOVEM-		**Novemlobate,** having nine lobes
DEC(I)-	ten	**Decigram** (des'ig-ram), one-tenth of a gram
DEC(A)-		**Decanormal** (dek-ah-nor'mal), having ten times the strength of normal
CENT-	hundred	**Centigrade** (sen'ti-grad), having one hundred degrees
HECT(O)-		**Hectogram,** one hundred grams
MILL(I)-	thousand	**Millimeter,** a thousandth part of a meter
KIL(O)-		**Kilometer,** one thousand meters (meter is 39.37 inches)
DEMI-	half	**Demilune,** a half-moon formation
SEMI-		**Semiconscious,** half (or part) conscious
HEMI-		**Hemiplegia,** half-paralyzed (paralysis on one side)
SESQUI-	one and one-half	**Sesquihora,** an hour and one-half
EQUI-	equal	**Equilibrium,** equal balance
MULTI-	many	**Multipara** (mul-tip'arah), a woman who has borne more than one child
POLY-		**Polychromatic,** many-colored

Pseudo-Prefix	Meaning	Example
SUPER-	more; too many (excessive)	**Supernumerary,** more than the normal number
PER-		**Pertussis,** excessive coughing
HYPER-		**Hypertrophy** (hi-per'trof-e), excessive growth
EXTRA-		**Extrasystole** (ex-trah-sis'to-le), an additional contraction of the heart
SUB-	less (deficient)	**Subnormal,** less than normal
HYPO-		**Hypotension,** less than normal (low blood pressure)

PSEUDO-PREFIXES DENOTING COLOR

Pseudo-Prefix	Meaning	Example
CHROMA-	color	**Chromhidrosis,** colored sweat
ALBUMIN-	white	**Albuminuria,** albumin (white) in the urine
ALB-		**Albino,** a person with congenital absence of pigment in skin, hair and eyes
LEUC-		**Leucotoxic,** destructive to white blood cells
LEUK-		**Leukemia,** excess of white cells in the blood
AMAUR-	dark	**Amaurosis** (am-aw-ro'sis), darkness (blindness)
AURE-	golden	**Aurantiasis,** golden-yellow discoloration of skin

Pseudo-Prefix	Meaning	Example
CINER-	gray	**Cinerea,** the gray matter of the nervous system
POLIO-		**Poliomyelitis,** inflammation of the gray matter
CHLOR-	green	**Chloroma,** green tumor
GLAUC-		**Glaucoma,** eye disease in which the appearance of the eye was anciently likened to the "silver-green scales of the deep-sea fish"
VERDIN		**Verdohemin,** bile pigment in blood
CIRRH-	yellow	**Cirrhosis** (sir-o'sis) (of the liver, a condition in which the liver is fibrosed and often a tawny yellow)
LUTEIN-		**Luteinization,** process taking place at the site of a ruptured Graafian follicle
XANTH-		**Xanthodont,** a yellow tooth
CYAN-	blue	**Cyanosis,** blueness of the skin
INDIGO-		**Indigouria,** presence of indigo in urine
RUBE-	red	**Rubella,** German measles (rash is red)
ERYTHR-		**Erythrocyte,** red blood cell
MELAN-	black	**Melanemesis,** black vomit
PURPUR-	purple	**Purpuriferous,** producing purple pigment

Pseudo-Prefix	Meaning	Example
PORPHYR-	purple	**Porphyruria** (por-fir-u're-ah), purple-colored urine

PSEUDO-PREFIXES DENOTING POSITION

Pseudo-Prefix	Meaning	Example
ANTER (O) -	in front of	**Anteromedian** (an"te-ro-me'de-an), situated in front near the middle
DEXTR (O) -	to the right of	**Dextrocardia,** heart located in the right side of the chest
LATER (O) -	to the side of	**Lateroposition,** displacement to one side
LEV (O) -	to the left of	**Levophobia,** fear of things on the left
SINISTR (O) -		**Sinistrocerebral** (sin"is-tro-ser'e-bral), on the left side of the brain
MES-	in the middle of	**Mesosternum,** middle of the sternum
MEDI-		**Median,** situated in the middle
OPISTH-	backward	**Opisthotonos,** a condition in which the body is arched backward
POSTER (O) -	behind	**Posterolateral,** behind at the side

MISCELLANEOUS PSEUDO-PREFIXES

Pseudo-Prefix	Meaning	Example
ACR (O) -	extremity	**Acromion process,** the tip of the shoulder blade

Pseudo-Prefix	Meaning	Example
AMBLY-	dim	**Amblyopia,** dimness of vision
ANDR-	man	**Android,** shaped like a man
ANISO-	unequal	**Anisopia,** inequality of vision in the two eyes
ATEL(O)-	imperfect	**Atelectasis,** imperfect expansion (of the lungs)
BLAST-	germ	**Blastomycosis,** a condition caused by fungus
BRACHY-	short	**Brachycephalic,** having a short head
BRADY-	slow	**Bradycardia,** a slow heartbeat
CRY-	cold	**Cryosurgery,** destruction of tissue by extreme cold
CRYM-		**Crymotherapy,** treatment by the application of cold
CRYPT(O)-	hidden	**Cryptorchidism** (krip-tor'kid-izm), a condition in which the testicles have not descended into the scrotum
CYT-	cell	**Cytoid,** resembling a cell
DOLICHO-	long	**Dolichocephalous,** having a long head
FIBR-	ropelike or like fiber	**Fibroma,** a tumor containing fibrous tissue
GYMNO-	naked	**Gymnophobia,** morbid dislike to the sight of nakedness

Pseudo-Prefix	Meaning	Example
GYN-	woman	**Gynecology** (jin-e-kol'o-je), the study of diseases peculiar to women
HETERO-	different or other	**Heterotropia,** a difference in the movement of the two eyes
		Heteroplasm, tissue not normal to a part
HIST-	weblike	**Histology,** the study of tissues
HYDR-	water	**Hydrotherapy,** treatment by the use of water
IATR-	physician	**Iatrogenic,** diseases (those produced by a physician)
IDIO-	one's own	**Idiopathic,** self-originated
IS-	equal	**Isotonic,** of equal tension
JUXTA-	adjoining	**Juxta-articular** (juks"tah-ar-tik'u-lar), near a joint
LEIO-	smooth	**Leiomyoma** (li"o-mi-o'mah), smooth muscle tumor
LEPTO-	thin	**Leptophonia,** a weak voice
LITH-	stone	**Lithotripsy,** crushing of a stone
MACR-	great	**Macrocheilia** (mac-ro-ki'le-ah), having abnormally large lips
MEGA-		**Megadontia,** having abnormally large teeth
MEGAL-		**Megalomania,** madness with illusions of greatness

Pseudo-Prefix	Meaning	Example
MER-	part	**Meropia,** partial blindness
MICR-	small	**Microscope,** an instrument for viewing small things
MORPH-	form	**Morphology,** the study of structures
MYC-	fungus	**Mycosis,** a condition in which a fungus is present
NARC-	numbness	**Narcotic,** an agent inducing deep sleep
NE(O)-	new	**Neoplasm,** new growth or tumor
OLIG-	few	**Oliguria,** scanty output of urine
ONC-	tumor	**Onchotherapy,** treatment of tumors
ORTH-	straight	**Orthopedist,** originally one who straightened the deformities of children
OXY-	sharp	**Oxycephalic,** having a sharply-pointed head
PACHY-	thick	**Pachydermatous,** having a thick skin
PALEO-	old	**Paleogenetic,** not newly acquired
PAN-	all	**Pansinusitis,** inflammation of all sinuses
PHOT-	light	**Photophobia,** fear of light
PLATY-	broad	**Platycephalic,** having a broad (wide) head

Pseudo-Prefix	Meaning	Example
PROT(O)-	first	**Protoplasm,** the first thing formed, e.g., primary substance of the embryo
PSEUD(O)-	false	**Pseudocyesis,** false pregnancy
PY(O)-	pus	**Pyorrhea,** a flow of pus
SAPRO-	decayed	**Saprodontia,** decayed teeth
SARC(O)-	flesh	**Sarcomyces,** fleshy fungus growth
SCIRRH-	hard	**Scirrhosarca** (skir-o-sark'ah), hardened tissue or skin
SCLER-		**Sclerosing,** causing or undergoing a process of hardening
SCOLIO-	curved or crooked	**Scoliosis,** curvature of the spine
SOMAT-	body	**Somatomegaly,** gigantism
STEN-	contracted	**Stenocardia,** narrowing of the coronary arteries of the heart
STEREO-	solid	**Stereoscopic,** giving a solid appearance to objects viewed
TACHY-	fast	**Tachycardia,** a fast heartbeat
THERM-	heat	**Thermometer,** an instrument for measuring temperature, i.e., heat

Pseudo-Prefix	Meaning	Example
TOXI-	poison	**Toxicology,** the study of poisons
TROPH-	nourishment	**Trophedema,** swelling of a part due to altered nourishment of it
VAS-	vessel	**Vasospasm,** spasm of the blood vessels

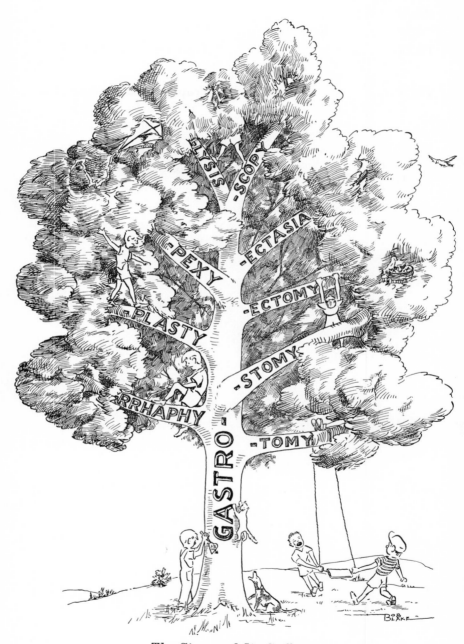

The Stem and Its Suffixes

Chapter V

SUFFIXES AND PSEUDO-SUFFIXES

A SUFFIX is a letter or syllable at the end of a word. Its function is much the same as that of the prefix. It also adds to a meaning. For example: *ist* as in the word "optimist" (one who practices optimism) or as in the word "fascist" (one who practices fascism) ; orthopedist (one who practices medicine in Orothopedics). Examples such as these may be called true suffixes, and while there are many of these, there are still many more of the pseudo type.

Instruction in suffixes may be by the same method used in teaching and learning prefixes.

PART I

SUFFIXES DENOTING RELATION, CONDITION, ABILITY

Suffix	*Meaning*	*Example of Use*
-ABLE	ability	**Potable,** capable of being drunk safely
-IBLE		**Digestible,** capable of being digested
-AL	related to	**Prodromal,** relating to the pre-onset stage of illness
-AC		**Cardiac,** relating to the heart or the cardia of the stomach
-IOUS		**Contagious,** communicable by touch
-IC		**Pyloric,** relating to the pylorus
-EAL	of that kind	**Lacteal,** milky

[43]

Suffix	Meaning	Example of Use
-EOUS	of that kind	**Calcareous,** chalky
-OSE		**Adipose,** fat
-OUS		**Bulbous,** bulblike
-IA	condition	**Anemia,** the condition of bloodlessness
-IASIS		**Cholelithiasis,** stones in bile passages
-ID		**Flaccid,** the condition of being soft
-ISM		**Mutism,** the condition of being mute
-OSIS		**Tuberculosis,** the condition of infection by the bacillus tuberculosis
-TION		**Constipation,** the condition of being constipated
-Y		**Apoplexy,** the condition of having suffered a stroke
-IST	agent (one who practices)	**Allergist,** one skilled in the treatment of allergies
-OR		**Operator,** one who operates
-ER		**Examiner,** one who examines
-ICIAN		**Physician,** one skilled in the practice of medicine
-ITY	quality	**Visibility,** the quality of being visible
-IUM	miniature or diminutive	**Manubrium,** a little handle (upper part of sternum)
-OLUS		**Gladiolus,** a little sword (middle part of sternum)
-OLUM		**Hordeolum,** a little grain of barley (description for a stye)
-CULUS		**Homunculus,** a little man (a word common in psychiatry)

Suffix	Meaning	Example of Use
-CULUM		**Diverticulum,** a little byway
-CLE		**Tubercle,** a little knot or knob
-CULE		**Molecule,** a little mass
-IZE	act in a certain way	**Catheterize,** to pass a catheter
-OMA	a new growth or tumor	**Carcinoma,** a cancerous growth (plural of oma is *omata,* as in fibromyomata; however, modern writers will write carcinomas.)

MISCELLANEOUS PSEUDO-SUFFIXES

Pseudo-Suffix	Meaning	Example
-AGO	disease	**Lumbago,** lumbar disease
-IGO	(old Latin)	**Impetigo,** (impetere = to attack) an acute inflammatory skin disease
-AGRA	rough	**Pellagra,** (pellis = skin) a disease characterized by rough skin
-ALGIA	pain	**Neuralgia,** nerve pain
-ATRESIA	without opening	**Proctatresia,** imperforate anus
-BLAST	germ	**Myeloblast,** an immature bone marrow cell
-CELE	swelling	**Hydrocele,** a collection of fluid in the *tunica vaginalis* of the testis
-CIDE	a killer	**Bactericide,** an agent which kills bacteria

Pseudo-Suffix	Meaning	Example
-CLEISIS	a closure	**Enterocleisis** (en-ter-o-kli'sis), a closure of the intestine
-CLYSIS	injection	**Enteroclysis** (en-ter-ok'lis-is), injection of nourishment into the bowel
-COCCUS	spherical bacterium (orig., a berry)	**Pneumococcus,** a bacterium of pneumonia
-CYST	sac of fluid	**Dacrocyst,** tear duct
-CYTE	cell	**Leukocyte,** a white blood cell
-DYNIA	pain	**Pleurodynia,** pain in the side (the pleura)
-ECTASIA	expansion	**Proctectasia,** dilatation of the anus
-ECTASIS	expansion	**Atelectasis,** imperfect expansion of the lung
-EMESIS	vomiting	**Hyperemesis,** excessive vomiting
-EMIA	of the blood	**Anemia,** bloodlessness
-ESTHESIA	sensation	**Anesthesia,** absence of sensation
-FORM	shape	**Ensiform,** sword-shaped
-FUGE	expeller	**Vermifuge,** an agent which expels worms from the body
-GENESIS	production	**Osteogenesis** (os"te-o-jen'es-is), bone development or production
-GRAM	a writing	**Electrocardiogram** (E.K.G.), a record of the heart's action made by an electrocardiograph

Pseudo-Suffix	Meaning	Example
-GRAPHY	writing	**Encephalography,** examination of the brain
-ITIS	inflammation	**Appendicitis,** inflammation of the vermiform appendix
-LITH	stone	**Nephrolith,** stone in the kidney
-LOGY	study of	**Pathology,** study of disease
-MALACIA	softening	**Osteomalacia,** softening of bone
-MANIA	madness	**Dipsomania,** pathological drinking of alcoholic beverages
-METER	measure	**Thermometer,** an instrument for measuring temperature
-OID	resembling	**Typhoid,** resembling typhus
-OPIA	vision	**Diplopia,** double vision
-OREXIA	appetite	**Anorexia,** loss of appetite
-PAROUS	bearing	**Multiparous,** having borne more than one child
-PATHY	disease	**Adenopathy,** disease of a gland
-PENIA	poor	**Thrombopenia,** decrease in number of blood platelets
-PHYLAXIS	a guarding	**Prophylaxis,** measures preventing the development or spread of disease
-PHYMA	growth or thickening	**Rhinophyma,** swelling and thickening of nose
-PHYTE	plant; fungus	**Dermatophyte,** skin fungus

Pseudo-Suffix	Meaning	Example
-PLASIA	formation	**Achondroplasia,** failure of cartilage to form at ends of long bones
-PNEA	breathing	**Dyspnea,** difficult breathing
-PTOSIS	a falling	**Gastroptosis** (gas-tro-to'sis), a falling of the stomach
-(R)RHAGE	a bursting forth	**Hemorrhage,** flow of blood
-(R)RHAGIA	a bursting forth	**Metrorrhagia,** uterine hemorrhage independent of the menstrual period
-(R)RHEA	a flow	**Diarrhea,** (a flow through) a condition characterized by increased frequency and lessened consistency of the fecal evacuations (bowel movements)
-(R)RHEXIS	rupture	**Gastrorrhexis,** rupture of the stomach
-SPASM	contraction	**Laryngospasm,** contraction of the vocal cords
-STASIS	position	**Metastasis** (met-as'tas-is), change of position (e.g., a manifestation of cancer at a site distant from its origin)
-STAXIS	discharge by drops	**Epistaxis,** nosebleed
-STHEN	strength	**Neurasthenia,** debility of the nerve centers
-THERAPY	treatment	**Radiotherapy,** treatment by the use of radium
-TROPHY	nourishment	**Dystrophy,** faulty nourishment

Pseudo-Suffix	Meaning	Example
-TROPIC	a turning	**Ectropic,** turned out, everted
-URIA	in the urine	**Hematuria,** blood in the urine

PART II

SUFFIXES, WORDS AND PHRASES ON OPERATIVE TERMINOLOGY[1]

Operations are classified in nine groups of procedures in the Standard Nomenclature of Operations, as follows:

0. *Incision*
1. *Excision*
2. *Amputation*
3. *Introduction*
4. *Endoscopy* (en-dos′ko-pe)
5. *Repair*
6. *Destruction*
7. *Suturing*
8. *Manipulation*

In these classifications are given suffixes as well as *complete phrases, words* and *synonymous terms* on operative procedure. In learning and reviewing these terms, the student may be helped considerably to interpret correctly words used by the surgeons in naming and describing operations.

These nine procedures are examined below.

0 — *Incision* (*cutting into; opening*)

The suffixes commonly employed for operations consisting of incisions are:

-(O)TOMY	(Gr. *tome* = a cutting)
-(O)STOMY	(Gr. *stoma* = a mouth)
-CENTESIS	(Gr. *kentesis* = puncture)

---

[1] *Standard Nomenclature of Diseases and Operations* (Chicago, Ill.: American Medical Association).

The procedures undertaken in this classification include:

Procedure	*Example*
-OTOMY (to cut into)	
Exploratory procedures	**Laparotomy** (Gr. *lapara* — the flank), opening the perito- neal cavity for exploratory purposes
Removal of foreign bodies	
(i) accidental	(i) **Removal of foreign body from eye**
(ii) therapeutic	(ii) **Removal of surgical nail, pin, screw, wire, etc.**
(iii) pathological	(iii) **Removal of calculi**
Divisions for investigation	**Partial transection of muscles, tendons, nerves, etc.**
Discission	**Needling of lens**
Decompression	**Craniotomy,** cutting or break- ing up the skull
Re-opening	**Re-opening** of old wound
-OSTOMY (to cut into to form an opening)	
Incision and drainage	**Incision and drainage of infections: abscesses; hematomata**
-CENTESIS (puncture or aspiration)	
Aspiration	**Aspiration,** of free fluid
Puncture	**Thoracentesis** (tho″rah-sen- te′sis), puncture of the thorax for the removal of fluid
Trephination	**Trephination** of cornea, re- moving a circular section from the summit of a conical cornea (Gr. *trypanon* = a gimlet)

1 — *Excision* (= *cutting out*)

The suffixes employed for operations of excision are:

-ECTOMY   (Gr. *ektome* = a cutting out)
-EXERESIS   (Gr. *exairesis* = removal)

Procedure   *Example*

-ECTOMY (to cut out or excise)
The excisions are divided into two types:

TYPE I (*Partial, Subtotal*)

Procedure	Example
Resection (*secare* = to cut)	**Subtotal gastrectomy,** excision of part of the stomach
Biopsy (*bios* = life; *opsis* = vision)	**Biopsy of lymph node,** removal of lymph node from living subject for examination
Guttering	**Of bone**
Saucerization	**Of bone**
Curettage (*curette* = a spoon-shaped instrument)	**Curettage of uterus,** scooping out of retained material

TYPE II (*Complete, Total*)

Procedure	Example
Radical excision (*radix* = a root)	**Mastectomy,** removal of breast entirely
Obliteration (*obliterare* = to efface)	**of varicose vein** (by closure of lumen)
Extirpation (*extirpare* = to root out)	**of tonsils**
Avulsion (*avellere* = to tear away)	**of fingernail, scalp**
Extraction (*trahere* = to draw)	**of cataract**
Enucleation (*nucleus,* diminutive of *nux* = nut)	**of eye** (removal, whole and clean)

Procedure	Example
Evisceration (*viscera* = the bowels)	**of eye** (sclera is left)
Epilation (*pilus* = a hair)	**of hair** (pulled out by the root)
Ablation (*ab* = from; *latus* = detached)	**of a tumor**

-EXERESIS (to strip out)

Removal by pulling out (stripping)	**Neuroexeresis,** stripping out of a nerve

2 — *Amputation* (*cutting off*)

No suffix is required for these procedures, which are as follows:

Procedure	Example
Disarticulation (*articulus* = a joint)	**of leg** (at a joint)
Dismemberment (*membrum* = a limb)	**of leg** (through a bone)

3 — *Introduction*

No suffix is required for operations in the introduction procedures:

Procedure	Example
Injections (*jacere* = to throw)	**of serum** **of air** **of radiopaque substance** **of dye** **of alcohol** **of oil**
Transfusions (*fundere* = to pour)	**of whole blood** **of plasma** **of serum**

Procedure	*Example*
Implantations (to place in)	**of radon**
Insertions	**of radium**
	of wire
	of metal nails, pins
	of collapsible bag
	of pack, tampon
	of catheter
	of rubber tubing, drains
	intubation tube

4 — Endoscopy (= to look within)

The suffix for this procedure is:

-SCOPY (*skopeo* = I view)

In this procedure an instrument (a scope) much like a periscope in a submarine is used. The following procedures are examples:

Procedure	*Site*
Anoscopy (a-nos′ko-pe)	**of anus**
Bronchoscopy	**of bronchus**
Cystoscopy	**of the urinary bladder**
Esophagoscopy	**of esophagus**
Gastroscopy	**of stomach**
Laryngoscopy	**of larynx**
Otoscopy	**of the external ear**
Peritoneoscopy	**of peritoneal cavity**
Proctoscopy	**of rectum**
Rhinoscopy	**of nose**
Thoracoscopy	**of chest**
Tracheoscopy	**of trachea**
Urethroscopy	**of the urethra**

Opportunity may be taken by the surgeon to combine with endoscopy one or more of the following procedures:

> Crushing
> Dilation
> Drainage
> Excision
> Injection
> Irrigation
> Removal

Example of combination terminology would be: *Bronchoscopy* with *excision* or *drainage* or with any of the above.

5 — *Repair (plastics = to form)*

The suffixes used for plastic operations are:

-PLASTY	(*plasso* = I form)
-(O)STOMY	(*stoma* = a mouth)
-DESIS	(*desis* = a binding)
-PEXY	(*pexis* = a fixing)

The following procedures come within the Plastic group:

Procedure	*Site*
-PLASTY (repair or reform)	**nose** (rhinoplasty)
Lengthen or shorten	**tendon**
Graft	**of skin**
	of bone
	of cartilage
	of fat
Attach or reattach	**nerves; tendons**
Advancement	**of eye muscles (for strabismus)**
Recessions	**of eye muscles (for strabismus)**
Open reductions	**of bone fractures and dislocations**

-OSTOMY (used in this category of plastic surgery for the purpose of joining together and forming permanent openings between two normally distinct spaces, e.g., if a piece of an intestine is removed, the normal procedure would be to sew the two cut ends together. This plastic repair, cut end to cut end, would be called enterostomy.)

Procedure	*Site*
Anastomosis	**Gastro-enterostomy**
-DESIS	
Fusion	**of a joint**
Stabilization	**Arthrodesis,** surgical stabilization of a joint
-PEXY	
Fixation	**Gastropexy** (of stomach)
Suspension	**Hysteropexy** (of uterus)

6 — *Destruction* (= *breaking down*)

The suffixes commonly employed for operations here are:

-CLASIS	(Gr. *klan* = to destroy)
-TRIPSY	(Gr. *tribein* = to crush)
-LYSIS	(Gr. *lyein* = to loosen)

The following procedures come within this group:

Procedure	*Example*
-CLASIS (to break down)	
Fracturing and re-fracturing	**Osteoclasis**
-TRIPSY (to crush)	
Crushing	**Neurotripsy** (of nerve)
-LYSIS (to free)	
Freeing (from adhesions)	**Enterolysis** (of intestine)

Also the following procedures, for which no suffixes are used, are of the destruction type:

Procedure	*Example*
Cauterization (*kauterion* = a branding iron)	**sealing off of bleeding points by heat**
Fulguration (ful-gu-ra′shun) (*fulgur* = lightning)	**destruction of ulcerated tissue by electricity**
Debridement (da-bred-maw′)	**cleaning out of dirty wounds or lacerations**
Diathermy (*dia* = through; *thermos* = heat)	**heating cells of tissues almost to point of destruction**

7 — *Suturing* (= *sewing or suturing*)

The suffix used for suturing operations is:

-(R)RHAPHY   (Gr. *rhaphe* = a seam)

The following are procedures in which the suffix is used:

Procedure	*Site*
Capsulorrhaphy	**suturing of a joint capsule**
Myorrhaphy (mi-or′af-e)	**of muscle**
Tenorrhaphy	**of tendon**
Fasciorrhaphy	**of fascia**
Aponeurorrhaphy	**of aponeurosis**
Laryngorrhaphy	**of larynx**
Tracheorrhaphy	**of trachea**
Bronchorrhaphy	**of bronchus**
Cardiorrhaphy	**of heart**
Pericardiorrhaphy	**of pericardium**
Arteriorrhaphy	**of artery**
Phleborrhaphy	**of vein**
Aneurysmorrhaphy	**of aneurysm**

Procedure	*Site*
Glossorrhaphy	**of tongue**
Gastrorrhaphy	**of stomach**
Enterorrhaphy	**of intestine**
Duodenorrhaphy	**of duodenum**
Jejunorrhaphy	**of jejunum**
Proctorrhaphy	**of rectum**
Hepatorrhaphy	**of liver**
Choledochorrhaphy	**of bile ducts**
Cholecystorrhaphy	**of gallbladder**
Herniorrhaphy	**of hernia**
Nephrorrhaphy	**of kidney**
Ureterorrhaphy	**of ureter**
Cystorrhaphy	**of urinary bladder**
Urethrorrhaphy	**of urethra**
Episiorrhaphy	**of vulva**
Episioperineorrhaphy	**of vulva and perineum**
Colporrhaphy	**of vagina**
Colpoperineorrhaphy	**of vagina and perineum**
Hysterorrhaphy	**of uterus**
Oophororrhaphy	**of ovary**
Trachelorrhaphy	**of cervix uteri**
Perineorrhaphy	**of perineum**
Neurorrhaphy	**of nerve**

Material used for suturing includes:

Catgut
Horsehair
Silkworm
Linen
Metal clips

8 — *Manipulation* (= *handling*)

The suffixes used for operations of the manipulative type are:

-TASIS	(Gr. *tasis* = a stretching)
-ECTASIA	(Gr. *ek* = out,
	tasis = a stretched con-
	dition or dilatation)

The following are procedures in which these suffixes are used:

Procedure	*Example*
-TASIS	
Stretching	**Myotasis** (of muscle)
-ECTASIA	
Dilatation	**Gastrectasia** (of stomach)

Other procedures here are:

Procedure	*Example*
Closed reduction	**of bone fracture**
Application	**of plaster cast**

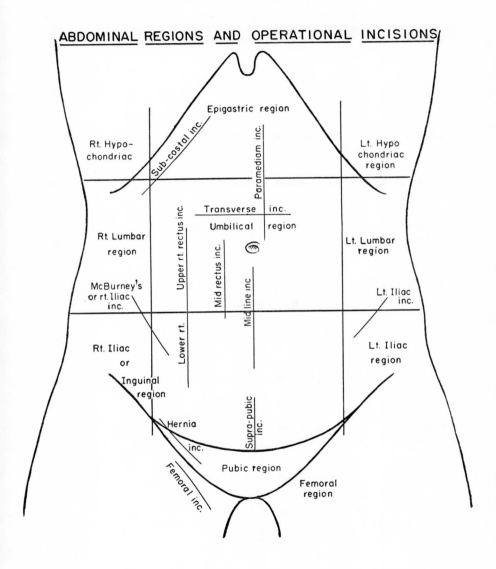

ABDOMINAL REGIONS AND OPERATIONAL INCISIONS

SURGICAL POSTURES

SURGICAL POSTURE IS OF SUFFICIENT IMPORTANCE TO WARRANT ITS INCLUSION ON THE RECORD OF OPERATION. SOME OF THE COMMON EXPRESSIONS FOUND IN OPERATIVE NOTES WHICH DESCRIBE POSTURES ARE SHOWN BELOW, WITH AN EXPLANATORY SYMBOLIC SKETCH.

POSTURE	SYMBOL	POSTURE	SYMBOL
DORSAL		PRONE	
RIGHT LATERAL		LEFT LATERAL	
HEAD RAISED FOWLER		HEAD LOWERED SCULTETUS	
HIGH PELVIC TRENDELENBURG		LITHOTOMY	
VERTICAL		DORSAL RECUMBENT	
ELLIOTT		DORSAL ELEVATED	
ROBSON		JACK-KNIFE	
THYROID		EDEBOHLS	
GALL BLADDER		LEFT SEMI-PRONE	
RIGHT KIDNEY		LEFT KIDNEY	

CHAPTER VI

MEDICAL WORD STEMS

IN THE preface of *Gould's Medical Dictionary,* Fifth Revised Edition, you will read that medical terminology "is made up of the unchanged and undigested materials and relics used or contributed during its entire history. . . . The result is a strange hodge-podge of medical language of two or more thousand years and of many special national tongues . . . with modern sounds and symbols, the whole amazingly heterogenous and cacophonous."

Discouraging as this description may be, the determined student can attain a working comprehension of medical word meanings without the aid of either history or philology, and the method is simple enough, granted the student has certain qualities. These qualities are: the ability to analyze words and try forms in re-use; the will to look things up; and the gift of memorizing. The student who can identify the constituent parts of a newly encountered word, who is willing to reach for a medical dictionary to hunt up a hitherto unmet component, try it out in another use, and is able to memorize its meaning, will soon become articulate in medical language. To the extent that these qualities are lacking, the student will be slow in attaining fluency, or may even fail altogether. This is because the task set is that of mastering a vocabulary rather than learning a tongue.

Medical words are, for the most part, names; often clumsy, often made polysyllabic by being hung fore and aft with *affixes*[1] of various kinds, but still merely names. Verbs and other essential parts of speech do occur, but not in large numbers. Many of the words are sad barbarisms. There is no grammar, no orderly arrangement in medical terminology, no question of maintaining

---

[1] Affix: either a prefix or suffix.

a conversation in medical words exclusively. Observe the proportion of plain English in the following extract from a (mythical) hospital record:

"Simple mastoidectomy. Nitrous oxide-ether anesthetic. Incision over the mastoid showed tissues to be highly congested. The bleeding was very free. Cortex was removed with gouge and rongeur. Mastoid cells had all broken down, and there was free pus found throughout. The sinus was uncapped by the infection for a space of one-half inch in the lower part. Bone necrosis extended up into the zygoma. With a curette, the necrotic bone was thoroughly cleaned, and the antrum, which contained a few granulations, was lightly curetted. The cavity was packed with iodoform gauze, bringing one end out at the tip. The wound was closed with dermal. Patient left the table in a very good condition."

In the operation report just quoted, no fewer than 75 per cent of the words employed are ordinary English words; better still, they are short English words. The medical words here are almost all the names of anatomical parts, instruments or dressings.

The basic component of any medical word is a STEM, or it may be called the body of a word; the supporting part. Exceptionally, the stem may be of Arabic, Anglo-Saxon, French, German, Dutch, or other — even Sanskrit — origin.

It follows that the task of mastering the medical vocabulary will be greatly helped if the student knows a stem, even a strange one, when he sees it, even though he is not versed in ancient or modern languages. He can do this best if he possesses, in his memory, a stock of these stems and their meanings, so that having identified a syllable in a long word as a stem, he may mentally check whether it is an old friend or a new one.

Clearly, a means of identifying medical word stems is the student's prime need. An excellent means of identifying them was given, by inference, more than 90 years ago in F. R. Campbell's *Language of Medicine*. Campbell defined a stem as "that part of a word which remains after the prefixes, suffixes and inflectional endings have been removed; or, rather, the part to which these affixes are added." As will be seen later, more than one stem is employed in many words, but, in short, Campbell said, "Take away the trimmings and behold: the stem." For example:

PROGNOSIS (a forecast)

divides into

PRO-   GNOSIS

(Prefix meaning *before*)   (Stem meaning *knowledge*)

The detection of stems by Campbell's method of subtraction requires the student to be familiar with affixes. The following is a *minimal* list of stems in which the modern meanings have been amplified descriptively where necessary. This list has been arranged according to the topographical classification of the Standard Nomenclature of Diseases.

SYSTEM 0 — BODY AS A WHOLE

Stem	*Modern Meaning*	*Example of Use*
BIOS	LIFE	**Biochemics,** the chemistry of life
EPIPLOON	OMENTUM (a fold of the peritoneum connecting the abdominal viscera to the stomach)	**Epiplocele,** a hernia containing omentum
MEDIAS-TINUM	MEDIASTINUM	**Mediastinitis,** inflammation of the mediastinum (me"de-as-ti'num)
PSYCHE	MIND	**Psychosis,** any morbid mental state
SARC	FLESH	**Sarcoid,** resembling flesh
TEINEIN	PERITONEUM (the serous membrane lining the abdominal cavity and enclosing the viscera)	**Retroperitoneal abscess,** an abscess behind the peritoneum

SYSTEM 1 — INTEGUMENTARY[1]

Stem	Modern Meaning	Example of Use
CUTIS	SKIN	**Subcutaneous,** under the skin
DERMA	SKIN	**Epidermis,** the outer layer of the skin
DIAPHOREO	PERSPIRATION	**Diaphoretic,** causing perspiration
GALACT	MILK	**Galactedema,** a swelling of the breast due to an accumulation of milk within it
MAMMA	BREAST	**Mammary gland**
MASTOS	BREAST	**Mastopexy,** surgical fixation of a pendulous breast
ONYCHIA	NAIL	**Onychophyma,** thickening of nails
PAPILLA	NIPPLE	**Papillate,** shaped like a nipple
PILUS	HAIR	**Pilous,** hairy
THEL	NIPPLE	**Thelalgia,** pain in the nipple
TRICHOS	HAIR	**Trichatrophia,** a brittle state of the hair from atrophy of the hair-bulbs

SYSTEM 2 — MUSCULOSKELETAL

Stem	Modern Meaning	Example of Use
ARTHRON	JOINT	**Synarthrosis,** an immovable joint

---

[1]Integumentary (*in* = in; *tegere* = to cover): covering of body; the skin.

Stem	Modern Meaning	Example of Use
BURSA	BURSA (a small sac between moving parts)	**Bursiform,** resembling a bursa or purse
CARPUS	WRIST	**Metacarpal,** pertaining to that part of the hand between the wrist and the fingers
CEPHALE	HEAD	**Dicephalous,** two-headed
CHEIR or CHIR	HAND	**Chirospasm** (ki'ro-spazm), writer's cramp
CHONDROS	CARTILAGE	**Achondroplasia,** lack of development of cartilage
COCCYX	COCCYX (last bone of spinal column)	**Coccygodynia** (kok"sig-o-din'e-ah), pain in the coccygeal region
COSTA	RIB	**Intercostal,** between the ribs
COXA	HIP	**Coxalgia,** pain in the hip
DACTYLOS	FINGER	**Dactylogram** (dak-til'o-gram), a fingerprint
DESMO	LIGAMENT	**Desmotomy,** division of ligaments
DIAPHRAG-MA	DIAPHRAGM (the sheet of muscle separating the thoracic and abdominal cavities)	**Diaphragmatic hernia,** a protrusion of some part of the abdominal viscera into the thorax through the diaphragm
KINESIS	MOVEMENT	**Kinetocyte,** a wandering cell
KRANION	SKULL	**Cranioplasty,** surgical repair of the skull
MUSCULUS	MUSCLE	**Intramuscular,** within the muscle

Stem	Modern Meaning	Example of Use
MYELOS	MARROW	**Myelatrophy,** wasting of the spinal cord
MY(O)	MUSCLE	**Myocarditis,** inflammation of the heart muscle
MYXA	MUCUS	**Myxorrhea,** a copious mucous flow
OMOS	SHOULDER	**Omodynia,** pain in the shoulder
OSTEON	BONE	**Osteomalacia,** softening of bone
PERONE	FIBULA	The **peroneal artery** supplies the muscles and integument of leg and foot
PES	FOOT	**Talipes,** clubfoot
POD	FOOT	**Podiatrist,** one who treats the foot (a chiropodist)
SPONDY-LOS	VERTEBRA (spinal bone)	**Spondylitis,** inflammation in a vertebral joint
TENON	TENDON	**Tenotomy,** the cutting of a tendon

SYSTEM 3 — RESPIRATORY

Stem	Modern Meaning	Example of Use
BRONCH	BRONCHUS (air tube to the lungs)	**Bronchoscope,** an instrument for viewing the interior of the bronchus
PECTUS	CHEST	**Pectoriloquy,** the voice heard through the chest
PHREN	DIAPHRAGM (sheet of muscle separating the thoracic and abdominal cavities)	**Phrenocostal,** pertaining to the diaphragm or the ribs

Stem	Modern Meaning	Example of Use
PNEUMON	LUNG	**Pneumonia,** inflammation of the lung
RHIN	NOSE	**Rhinoplasty,** surgical repair of the nose
THORAX	CHEST	**Thoracentesis,** puncture of the thorax to remove fluid
TRACHEIA	WINDPIPE	**Tracheotomy,** surgical incision of the windpipe

SYSTEM 4 — CARDIOVASCULAR

Stem	Modern Meaning	Example of Use
ANGEION	VESSEL	**Angioma,** a tumor formed of small blood vessels
AORTE	AORTA	**Aortostenosis,** narrowing of the aorta
ARTERIA	ARTERY	**Arteriosclerosis,** chronic thickening of the arterial walls, which makes them appear hard
CARDIA	HEART	**Pericardium,** the membranous sac enclosing the heart
PHLEBO	VEIN	**Phlebotomy,** opening of a vein; to let blood
VENA	VEIN	**Venule,** small vein
SPHYGMOS	PULSE	**Sphygmomanometer** (sfig''-mo-man-om'et-er), an instrument for measuring pulse pressure, i.e., blood pressure

SYSTEM 5 — HEMIC & LYMPHATIC

Stem	Modern Meaning	Example of Use
ADEN	GLAND	**Adenoblast,** a gland cell
HEMA	BLOOD	**Hemophilia,** an abnormal tendency to bleed
SPLEN	SPLEEN	**Splenectomy,** removal of the spleen

SYSTEM 6 — DIGESTIVE

Stem	Modern Meaning	Example of Use
AMYGDALE	TONSIL	**Amygdaloid fossa** (almond-shaped fossa), the depression for the lodgement of the tonsil
CHEILOS	LIP	**Cheiloschisis** (ki-los′kis-is), harelip
CHOLE	BILE	**Cholelithotripsy,** crushing of a gallstone
CHYLOS	CHYLE (liquefied food passing from duodenum to intestine)	**Chyluria,** chyle in the urine
COLON	COLON (the large bowel)	**Colonic,** relating to the colon
COPROS	EXCREMENT	**Coprolith,** a hard mass, like a stone, of fecal matter in the bowels
DIPSA	THIRST	**Dipsomania,** uncontrollable desire for spirituous liquors
EMESIS	VOMITING	**Hematemesis** (hem-at-em′esis), vomiting of blood

Stem	Modern Meaning	Example of Use
ENTERON	GUT	**Enteric fever,** typhoid fever
GASTER	STOMACH	**Gastroscopy,** inspection of the interior of the stomach with an instrument
GLOSSA[1]	TONGUE	**Glossitis,** inflammation of the tongue
GLOTTIS	GLOTTIS (a part of the voice box)	**Glottal,** pertaining to the glottis
HEPATO	LIVER	**Hepatopexy,** surgical fixation of the liver
ILEOS	ILEUM (lower portion of the small intestine)	**Ileoparietal,** relating to the walls of the ileum
LARYNX	LARYNX (the throat)	**Laryngitis,** inflammation of the larynx
MESOS- ENTERON	MESENTERY (a peritoneal fold connecting the small intestine with the posterior abdominal wall)	**Mesenteroid,** pertaining to the mesentery
ODONT	TOOTH	**Odontodynia,** toothache
OISOPHA- GOS	GULLET (esophagus)	**Esophagoptosis,** falling of the gullet
OREXIS	APPETITE	**Anorexia,** absence of appetite
PHAGEIN	SWALLOWING	**Dysphagia,** difficulty in swallowing
PHARYNX	PHARYNX	**Pharyngeal,** pertaining to the pharynx

[1] Also lingua, e.g., lingual tonsils.

Stem	Modern Meaning	Example of Use
PROKTOS	ANUS or RECTUM	**Proctoscopy,** inspection of the rectum by an instrument
PYLOROS	PYLORUS (ring-like aperture between the stomach and duodenum)	**Pyloric stenosis,** stricture of the pylorus
STOMA	MOUTH	**Stomatitis,** inflammation of the mouth
TONSILLA	TONSIL	**Tonsillectomy,** surgical removal of the tonsils

SYSTEM 7 — UROGENITAL

Stem	Modern Meaning	Example of Use
COLPOS	VAGINA (canal leading to the uterus)	**Colpocele,** hernia into the vagina
CYSTIS	BLADDER	**Cystoma,** tumor of the bladder
DIDYMOI	EPIDIDYMIS (the small body lying above the testis)	**Epididymotomy,** cutting the epididymis
GENOS	GENESIS	**Genetics,** the laws of generation
HYMEN	HYMEN (membrane partly closing the vagina)	**Hymenorrhaphy,** suturing of the hymen
HYSTERA	WOMB/UTERUS	**Hysteromyoma,** a type of uterine tumor
KLEITORIS	CLITORIS (female homologue of the penis)	**Clitoridectomy,** excision of the clitoris

Stem	Modern Meaning	Example of Use
LOCHIOS	LOCHIA (the discharge following birth of a child)	**Lochiorrhagia,** an excessive flow of the lochia
METRA	WOMB/UTERUS	**Metritis,** inflammation of the uterus
NEPHROS	KIDNEY	**Hydronephrosis,** a collection of urine in the kidney pelvis
NYMPHE	NYMPHAE (the labia minora of the vulva)	**Nymphoncus** (nim-fong'-kus), a tumor or swelling of the nympha
OOPHO-REIN	OVARY (the egg-producing organ of the female)	**Oöphoropathy,** any disease of the ovary
ORCHIS	TESTICLE (the sperm-producing organ of the male)	**Cryptorchidism,** the retention of the testes in the abdomen or inguinal canal
PYELOS	KIDNEY PELVIS	**Pyelogram,** an X ray of the kidney pelvis and ureter
REN	KIDNEY	**Adrenal,** adjacent to the kidney
SALPINX	FALLOPIAN TUBE	**Salpingitis,** inflammation of the Fallopian tube
SPERMA	SEMEN (seed of the male)	**Spermicide,** a sperm-killer
TRACHEL	NECK (neck of uterus; or cervix)	**Trachelotomy,** cutting uterine neck
URINA	URINE	**Urinal,** a vessel for receiving urine

Stem	Modern Meaning	Example of Use
UTERUS	UTERUS	**Uterine gestation,** the carrying of a child in the womb
VESICULA	VESICLE (small bladder or sac-like structure)	**Vesiculiform** (ves-ik'u-li-form), shaped like a vesicle

SYSTEM 8 — ENDOCRINE

Stem	Modern Meaning	Example of Use
CAROTIS	CAROTID	**Carotid gland,** a ductless gland at the bifurcation of the common carotid artery
GONÊ	GONAD (a sexual gland, testis or ovary)	**Gonadotherapy,** use of gonadal extracts to correct or invigorate
PINEA	PINEAL (a ductless gland the secretions of which affect sex)	**Pinealectomy** (pin"e-al-ek'to-me), surgical removal of the pineal gland
PITUITA	PITUITARY (a ductless gland the secretion of which affects growth, maturity and many other things)	**Pituitrin** (pit-u'it-rin), a preparation made from the posterior lobe of the pituitary gland
THYMOS	THYMUS (ductless gland which normally atrophies after puberty)	**Thymusectomy,** excision of the thymus gland
THYREOS	THYROID (ductless gland the secretion of which is essential to the body's function)	**Hyperthyroidism,** excessive activity of the thyroid gland

SYSTEM 9 — NERVOUS

Stem	Modern Meaning	Example of Use
AESTHE-SIS	SENSATION	**Anesthesia,** absence of sensation
ENCEPHA-LOS	ENCEPHALON (Brain)	**Encephalitis,** inflammation of the brain
GANGLION	GANGLION (any collection or mass of nerve cells that serves as a center of nervous influence)	**Spinal ganglia,** those on the spinal nerve near the intervertebral foramina
GNOSIS	KNOWLEDGE	**Prognosis,** a forecast
LEPSIS	SEIZURE	**Epilepsy,** convulsive seizures
MENINX	MENINGES (membranes covering the brain and spinal cord)	**Meningitis,** inflammation of the membranes of the brain or spinal cord
MENS	MIND	**Dementia,** loss of mind
MNESIS	MEMORY	**Amnesia,** loss of memory
NEURON	NERVE	**Neuroma,** a tumor composed of nerve tissue
OPSIS	VISION	**Amblyopia ex anopsia,** dimness of vision due to disuse or nonuse
OSME	SMELL	**Anosmia,** absence of sense of smell
PATHOS	DISEASE	**Psychopath,** one ill in the mind
PHASIS	SPEECH	**Aphasia,** inability to articulate words or sentences

Stem	*Modern Meaning*	*Example of Use*
PHILIA	LIKING	**Necrophile,** one who violates dead bodies
PHOBOS	FEAR	**Claustrophobia,** fear of confined spaces
PHONÊ	VOICE	**Aphonia,** loss of voice

SYSTEM 10 — ORGANS OF SPECIAL SENSE

Stem	*Modern Meaning*	*Example of Use*
BLEPHA-RON	EYELID	**Blepharitis,** inflammation of the eyelids
PALPEBRA	EYELID	**Palpebrate,** to wink
CORÊ	PUPIL	**Coreometer,** an instrument for measuring the pupil of the eye
CORNEUS	CORNEA	**Corneal,** pertaining to the cornea
KERAS	CORNEA	**Keratocentesis,** puncture of the cornea
DACRYON	TEAR DUCT	**Dacrycystalgia** (dak″re-sis-tal′je-ah), pain in the lacrymal sac
IRIS	IRIS	**Iridodonesis,** a wavering of the iris
MYRINGA	EARDRUM	**Myringotomy,** incision of the tympanic membrane or eardrum
OPHTHAL-MOS	EYE	**Ophthalmia,** inflammation of eye
OTO	EAR	**Otitis,** inflammation of the ear

CHAPTER VII

SELECTED MEDICAL VOCABULARY

ON

1. Body Structures
2. Conditions of Body Structure
3. Diseases of Body Structure
4. Analysis of Words and Phrases
5. Narrations on Word Meanings
6. Definitions

IN THIS chapter we are dealing with concrete examples in medical terminology. The stems, prefixes and suffixes given in previous chapters are but steppingstones to provide a base for medical word mastery. The newcomer to the medical field will find that having learned these basic terms, he may be able to sally forth and make inroads on completed terms, full phrases and correct diction in the medical language.

Language derivations such as Greek, Latin, etc., are purposely omitted. It is felt that in such an elementary presentation the language derivation would but cause confusion, and any student having a desire to pursue such origins may do so through the references. Here we are dealing with systems of the body. Various examples of selected words and phrases are given under each anatomical system. The main considerations are:

1. Words or phrases used to denote the anatomical systems

2. Words or phrases to denote anatomical parts of each system

3. Words or phrases to name diseases (pathology) common to each system

4. Analysis of words (Analysis of a word means a division by component parts, showing the meaning of each part, and defining the word by combining the several meanings)

5. Narrations on origin of meaning

6. Definitions

Here, too, we have followed the general outline of systems as they are listed in *Standard Nomenclature of Disease.*[1] For reference on analysis and narrations and definitions, Dorland's *American Illustrated Medical Dictionary,*[2] *The Origin of Medical Terms*[3] by HENRY ALAN SKINNER, M.D., and *Medical Etymology*[2] by O. H. PERRY PEPPER, M.D., have been used.

Instruction in deciphering medical words and placing them in proper categories may be done in the following manner:

1. Pronounce the word — viz., my"o-kar-di'tis.

2. Spell the word.

3. Give analysis — viz., myo (muscle), cardia (heart), itis (inflammation of).

4. Define — viz., inflammation of heart muscle.

5. Name the anatomical system to which the word belongs — viz., cardiovascular system.

6. Name the specialist who may be concerned — viz., Cardiologist.

7. If the word indicates an operable disease, name the procedure.

PSYCHOBIOLOGICAL UNIT

(Specialist practicing in this field may be a Psychiatrist, Neurologist or Neuropsychiatrist)

PSYCHOBIOLOGICAL UNIT: (*psyche* = soul or mind; *bio* = life; *logos* = study of). That unit in the study of the human make-up which gives consideration to the influence of mind on life.

---

[1] American Medical Association, Chicago, Ill.

[2] W. B. Saunders Company, Philadelphia, Pa.

[3] Williams and Wilkins Company, Baltimore, Md.

ANALYSIS, DEFINITIONS AND NARRATIONS

Example Terms

DELIRIUM TREMENS: (*delirare* = to be crazy; from *lira* = furrow, hence, "off the track"; and *tremens* = trembling) shaking madness due to alcoholism.

DEPRESSIVE: (*premere* = to press down) causing a lowering of vitality.

HALLUCINOSIS: (*alucinari* = to wander in mind) a condition in which things are sensed which are nonexistent.

MANIC: (*mania*) frenzy.

PARESIS: (*paresis* = a letting go) general paralysis of the insane.

PSYCHOSIS: (*psyche* = mind; *osis* = condition of) a disordered condition of the mind.

SCHIZOPHRENIA: (*schizein* = to split; *phren* = mind) denoting dual personality (dementia praecox).

SENILITY: (*senescere* = to grow old; *senilis* = to grow old prematurely) pathologic aging.

BODY AS A WHOLE

BODY AS A WHOLE: Referring to diseases and conditions affecting the body generally.

ANALYSIS, DEFINITIONS AND NARRATIONS

Example Terms

ANTHRAX INFECTION: (*anthrax* = coal) an acute infection characterized by hot red skin lesions like "live coals."

BOTULISM: (*botulus* = a sausage) a disease caused by microorganisms in food.

PSITTACOSIS: (*psittakos* = a parrot) a disease of birds, especially parrots, which attacks man. It resembles a violent typhoid fever.

Example Terms

TETANUS: (*teinein* = to stretch) an infectious disease characterized by muscular spasms (lockjaw). It is caused by a bacillus, *Clostridium tetani.*

TETANY: (a derivative of the word tetanus) a condition characterized by intermittent spasms of the muscles, especially of the arms and hands. It is *not* caused by the bacillus of tetanus.

VACCINIA: (*vacca* = a cow) cowpox or the results of vaccination with the cowpox virus.

VITAMIN: (*vita* = life; *amin* = derived from ammonia) an organic compound present in natural foodstuffs. Different vitamins assist different physiological functions.

REGIONS

REGIONS: Localization to one section of the body.

ANALYSIS, DEFINITIONS AND NARRATIONS

Examples of Parts

MEDIASTINUM: (medial, intermediate, or between) the anatomical part denoting the space, fronted by the sternum, which contains: heart and pericardium, thoracic aorta and great vessels which arise from its arch, the pulmonary arteries, the great veins near the heart, and the remains of the thymus gland with lymph nodes and lymphatic vessels.

MESENCHYME: (*mesos* = middle; *enchyma* = infusion, or *en* = in; *chymos* = juice, or that which pours out) the word was first used in embryology to denote that part of the mesoderm which forms connective tissue. The term has been expanded to include other mesoderm derivatives.

OMENTUM: The origin of the term is not known. It is a duplication of the continuous layers of peritoneum leading from the stomach to nearby structures, such as the liver, etc.

PARIETAL PERITONEUM: (*paries* = wall; *peri* = around; *teinein* = stretched) a wall stretched around. In this instance it is the

Examples of Parts

lining of abdominal and pelvic walls. Peritoneum used alone refers only to abdominal wall lining.

PERINEUM: the origin of the word is obscure. It is the region between anus and scrotum in male, or region between anus and structures beginning at pelvic outlet in female.

SUPERFICIAL FOSSAE: (superficial = surface; *fossa* = ditch; plural is *fossae*). They are the external indentations or regional depressions, e.g., axilla, groin, etc.

UMBILICUS: (um-bil-i'kus) (*umbilicus* = navel). The Greek word for navel is *omphalos*. The word *umbo* means boss, a protuberant decorative part of a shield. The umbilicus is the scar which marks the site of entrance of the cord which feeds the child in utero.

INTEGUMENTARY SYSTEM

(Specialist practicing in this field is the Dermatologist)

INTEGUMENTARY SYSTEM: (*in* = in; *tegere* = to cover) that which covers; the skin covering the body.

ANATOMICAL PARTS

ANALYSIS, DEFINITIONS AND NARRATIONS

Example Terms

CILIA: (Plural of *cilium* = outer edge of eyelid) the eyelashes.

CORIUM: (leather) dermis or "true skin."

DERMIS: (*derma* = skin) layer of skin just beneath epidermis; called "true skin."

EPIDERMIS: (*epi* = on; *derma* = skin) outer layer of skin.

FOLLICLE: (*follis* = a bag; diminutive suffix, *cle*) a little bag. In the integumentary system this term is applied to hair follicles or pouches, from which springs the hair growth.

Example Terms

MUCOCUTANEOUS: (*muco* = referring to mucosa; *cutis* = skin) a membrane which is part mucosa and part skin.

MUCOUS MEMBRANE or MUCOSA: (*mucus* = watery secretion; *membrane* = lining). Any lining, secreting mucus, covering those canals and cavities which communicate with the external air.

NAIL BED: that part of corium upon which nail rests.

NAIL FOLDS: fold of tissue around base of nail.

PAPILLARY BODY: (*papilla* — pl. is *ae*) any small cone-shaped elevation. The small conical bodies or masses which project up into epidermis. They usually run in parallel lines and are the formations which, when reproduced, make fingerprints.

SEBACEOUS GLANDS: (*sebum* = tallow, suet or fat; *glans* = a secreting organ). A gland which produces a greasy substance.

STRATUM CORNEUM: (*stratum* = layer or blanket; *corneum* = horn-like or tough). Outermost horny layer of epidermis.

SUBCUTANEOUS: (*sub* = under; *cutis* = skin). Under the skin.

SUBCUTANEOUS AREOLAR TISSUE: (*sub* = under; *cutis* = skin; *areola* = area or courtyard, a diminutive area or a little open space). Loose connective tissue found under the skin; sometimes called *cellular tissue*.

SUDORIFEROUS GLANDS: (*sudor* = sweat; *ferre* = to bear). Glands which produce sweat.

CONDITIONS AND DISEASES OF INTEGUMENTARY SYSTEM

ANALYSIS, DEFINITIONS AND NARRATIONS

Example Terms

ACNE: (*achne* = chaff) any inflammatory condition of the sebaceous glands.

Example Terms

CARBUNCLE: (dimin. of *carbo* = hot coal) a reaction of the skin and subcutaneous tissue to an invasion by staphylococcal microorganisms, but more violent and over a larger area.

CHICKENPOX or VARICELLA: an acute contagious disease characterized by crops of superficial macules, papules and vesicles.

CICATRIX: the mark left by a lesion or wound; a scar. ("Lesion" is disease pathology, wound or local degeneration. "Sore" is sometimes used, but is non-medical terminology.)

DECUBITUS ULCERS: (*decumbere* = to lie down) large ulcerous areas or bedsores.

DERMATOPHYTOSIS: a fungus invasion of the skin; "athlete's foot."

DERMOID CYSTS: benign congenital cysts, which may contain embryonic tissue (viz., hair, skin and teeth).

EPIDERMOID CYSTS: benign cysts arising from displaced epidermal cells, usually on hands, forehead and top of head.

EROSION: (*e* = out; *rodere* = to gnaw) a dissolution or dying of the epidermis.

ERYSIPELAS: (perhaps *erythros* = red; *pella* = skin) reaction to streptococcal invasion (via a wound) of lymphatics of skin, or of mucous membranes.

EXCORIATION: (*ex* = out; *corium* = skin) any superficial loss of substance such as that produced by scratching.

FISSURE: (*fissura* = a cleft or slit) any cleft or groove in the skin. It generally extends into the corium.

FURUNCLE: (boil; literally, "little thief") an infection occurring without any pre-existing wound. It is the invasion of hair follicles by staphylococci (microorganisms), and if only one follicle is involved the lesion is called a furuncle.

GAS GANGRENE INFECTION: (*gangraina* = an eating sore or dying tissue) invasion of skin and muscles by gas bacillus carried by dirt, explosive powder and foreign bodies.

Example Terms

IMPETIGO: an inflammatory skin disease characterized by isolated pustules.

LEUKOPLAKIA: a disease characterized by white, thickened patches on inner cheek, gums, tongue, or any mucosa.

MACULE: (*macula* = a spot) a nonelevated discoloration.

MEASLES: a contagious eruptive fever characterized by dark pink macules.

MUCOUS CYSTS: cystically dilated mucous glands, following inflammation or injury.

MYCOSIS: (*mykes* = fungus; *osis* = a condition of) invasion of tissue by fungus growth.

PAPULE: (*papula* = a pimple) a hard elevated lesion.

PARONYCHIA: (*para* = beside; *onyx* = claw or nail) infection usually introduced through torn nail fold (hangnail); may also be called a "run-a-round."

PIGMENTATION: the deposition of coloring matter. It may result from sunlight, scratching, mustard plaster, tattooing, etc.

PSORIASIS: a skin disease characterized by scaly red patches on the skin.

PUSTULE: (*pus* = pus) an elevated lesion containing pus.

SCARLET FEVER: an acute contagious fever characterized by a scarlet eruption.

SMALLPOX or VARIOLA: an acute infectious disease characterized by an eruption which is progressively papular, vesicular, and pustular.

STEATOMA or SEBACEOUS CYST: cystic formation caused by retention of sebaceous gland substance; sometimes called "wen."

TROPHIC ULCER: (*trophe* = nourishment) large, necrotic areas due to lack of nourishment, e.g., from poor circulation.

Example Terms

ULCER: (*ulcus* = ulcer) an open lesion other than a wound. There are three types — punched out, undermining, and sloping.

VARICOSE ULCERS: a secondary result of varicose veins.

VESICLE: an elevated lesion containing fluid.

BREAST

ANALYSIS, DEFINITION AND NARRATIONS

Example Terms

INTERSTITIAL TISSUE: (*inter* = between; *sistere* = to stand) connective tissue between cells of an organ.

MAMMARY GLAND: (*mamma* = udder or breast). The word is said to be derived from "ma-ma," the cry of the infant — a first cry which is distinguishable in the infant in all languages and which in all countries is likely to indicate hunger in the child.

PARENCHYMATOUS TISSUE: (*para* = beside; *enchyma* = infusion or juice). This term originated when it was thought that materials of the blood were poured in the organs and there infused to form the substance of the organ. Gradually the term has come to mean infusion into cells of the organs. Parenchymatous tissue is that part of an organ which is essential, or the functional part.

MUSCULOSKELETAL SYSTEM

(The specialist practicing in this field is an Orthopedist or sometimes called an Orthopedic Surgeon)

ANALYSIS, DEFINITION AND NARRATIONS

Example Terms

MUSCLE: (*mus* = a mouse; *cle* = diminutive suffix) a mouse. This thought comes presumably from the manner in which the muscles ripple and move under the skin.

Example Terms

SKELETON: (*skeletos* = dried up). The word was originally used in reference to a mummy or dried-up body. The modern interpretation is dry bones.

BONES AND JOINTS

ANALYSIS, DEFINITIONS AND NARRATIONS

Example Terms

ACETABULUM: (*acetum* = vinegar) the cup-shaped part of the hip-joint which receives the head of the femur. In Roman days, it was thought to resemble a small vinegar cruet.

BURSA: (*bursa* = pouch, purse) a closed sac.

CARPAL BONES: (*karpos* = wrist) the several bones of the wrist. These are *scaphoid* (boat-shaped), *pisiform* (round like a pea), *semilunar* (half-moon), *os magnum* (the largest carpal bone), *trapezium* (diamond-shaped), *cuneiform* (wedge-shaped), *trapezoid* (similar to the trapezium, but smaller) and *unciform* (hook-shaped).

CERVICAL VERTEBRAE: (*cervix* = neck) the 7 bones of the neck.

CLAVICLE: (*clavis* = a key) the collarbone, supposed to resemble the key of an instrument.

CONDYLES: (*kondylos* = a knuckle) the rounded eminences at the articular surfaces of bones.

CORACOID PROCESS:[1] (*korax* = a raven) a curved body projection from upper edge of the scapula, supposed to resemble a raven's bill.

CORONOID PROCESS:[1] (*korone* = a crow) a projection at the head of the ulna.

DIAPHYSIS: (*dia* = through; *physis* = growth) that which grows through from end to end; the shaft of a long bone. It originally was applied to the ligaments of a joint. The shaft of a bone is the stabilized part between the two growing ends.

[1]Process: a slender projecting point.

Example Terms

DORSAL VERTEBRAE: (*dorsum* = back) the 12 thoracic vertebrae.

EPIPHYSIS: (*epi* = upon; *physis* = growth) the growing ends of a bone, which is cartilage before it ossifies and causes elongation.

ETHMOID: (*ethmos* = a sieve) a bone at the upper part of the nose between the two orbital bones; the part at the back of the nose is pierced with numerous holes, through which pass the nerves conveying the sense of smell.

FEMUR: (*femur* = thigh) the thigh bone, longest in the body.

FIBULA: (*figo* = I fasten; *fibula* = a clasp, nail, pin) the "brooch bone" which clasps, through its *malleolus* (little hammer), the tibia in place.

GLENOID PROCESS: (*glene* = a cavity) the hollow which receives the head of the humerus.

HUMERUS: (*umerus* = the shoulder bone; *omos* = the shoulder) the bone of the upper arm.

HYOID: (*hyoeides* = U-shaped) a bone at the root of the tongue, attached to the skull by ligaments.

ILIUM: (*ilis* = soft) the "bone of the soft parts," i.e., the flanks; the hip bone. Attempts have been made to link the name with the city Ilium (of the "topless towers"), i.e., Troy, the connection being the rampart function of the iliac crest and the like function of Troy's walls.

ISCHIUM: (*ischion* = hip joint) the "seat bone."

LAMINA: (*lamina* = a plate) the side of a vertebra sloping towards the spinous process.

LUMBAR VERTEBRAE: (*lumbus* = loin) the five largest, heaviest, lowest vertebrae.

MALAR: (*mala*) the cheek bone. (*Maxilla* is a diminutive of mala, the upper jawbone.)

Example Terms

MANDIBLE: (*mandere* = to chew) the lower jaw, which crushes food against the upper.

MENISCUS: (diminutive from *men* = moon) crescent-shaped or little moon-shaped. A little moon being the quarter-moon; it is described here as a *semilunar cartilage.*

METAPHYSIS: (*meta* = together; *physis* = growth) line of juncture of epiphysis and diaphysis on long bones.

NUCLEUS PULPOSUS: (*nucleus* = a diminutive term meaning "nut" or "kernel"; *pulpa* = flesh) a little nut or heart of a shell which is softish; a semifluid mass in the center of an intervertebral disk. *Intervertebral disks* are the layers of fibrocartilage between the vertebrae.

OCCIPITAL: (*ob* = against; *caput* = head) the bone at the back of the head.

OLECRANON PROCESS: (*olene* = elbow; *kranion* = head) a projection at the head of the ulna, contributing strong support to the articulation with the humerus.

PATELLA: (*patella* = little plate) the kneecap.

PELVIC BONES: These are a combination of bones forming a cavity-like structure. They comprise, in the front—the *pubis,* on the sides—inner bones of the hip (*ilia*), and in the back —the *sacrum* and *coccyx.*

PHALANGES: (*phalanx* = soldiers in close order) finger bones.

PUBIC BONE: (*pubes* = adult) front of the pelvic bone, in two parts which fuse at the beginning of adult age. The point of fusion is called *symphysis pubis.*

RADIUS: (*radius* = the spoke of a wheel) the straight rodlike bone on the "thumb side" of the forearm.

RIBS: (Anglo-Saxon = *ribb*) 12 pairs of bones forming the thoracic (chest) cage. There are 7 pairs of "true" ribs and 5 pairs of "false" ribs, and of the 5 false pairs, 2 are "floating."

Example Terms

SACRUM : (*sacer* = sacred) a large triangular bone between the hip bones. This bone was thought by the ancients to survive after death and form part of the body in the resurrection. Another story is that the bone was held sacred because it protected the organs usually offered in sacrifices.

SCAPULA: (*scapula* = shoulder blade; perhaps *skaptein* = to dig) the shoulder blade. Possibly the "dig" derivation is right, as the bone is spadelike.

SESAMOID BONES: (*sesame* = a plant producing nutlike seeds; *oid* = like). The tendons of muscles sometimes contain small bony nodules, especially where they pass a joint. Because these nodules resemble the sesame seed, they are called sesamoid bones. The term now means accessory bones.

SKULL: a word of uncertain origin; possibly Anglo-Saxon (*skuhl* = head) or Scandinavian (*skaal* = bowl). This "hollow globe of bone" contains 22 bones, 8 forming the cranium and 14 the face.

SPHENOID: (*sphen* = a wedge) the "butterfly bone," which articulates with all the other cranial bones and binds them together.

SPINE: (*spina* = a thorn) a thornlike process of bone; the backbone.

STERNUM: (*sternon* = the male chest or flat chest) the breast bone. Its three parts are the *manubrium* (little handle), the *gladiolus* (little sword — a gladiator was a swordsman, the flower *gladiolus* has swordlike leaves), and the *ensiform process* (*ensis* = a sword). The notches in the sternum receive the true ribs.

STYLOID PROCESS: (*stylos* = a pillar) a bony projection at the lower extremity of the ulna.

SYMPHYSIS: (*syn* or *sym* = with; *physis* = growth) a growing together or a union. It is not a true joint.

Example Terms

TARSAL BONES: (*tarsos* = a wickerwork frame) the bones of the ankle. These are *calcaneus* or *os calcis* (*calx* = heel), *astragalus* (ankle bone), *cuboid* (cube-shaped), *navicular* (boat-shaped), *outer, middle* and *inner cuneiform* (wedge-shaped).

TEMPORAL: (*tempus* = time) the "time bone"; the "vital spot." It is over the temples that the hair first turns gray, indicating the passing of time.

TIBIA: the shin bone.

TROCHANTERS: (*trochos* = a wheel) eminences at the upper end of the femur, to which are attached the rotator muscles of the thigh.

ULNA: large inner bone of forearm.

VERTEBRA: (*vertere* = to turn) a turning joint. One of the 33 bones of the spine. The vertebrae comprise 7 cervical, 12 thoracic or dorsal, 5 lumbar, 5 sacral, and 4 coccygeal.

VOMER: (*vomer* = ploughshare) a thin plate of bone "ploughing" between the nostrils.

ZYGOMATIC ARCH: (*zygos* = yoke) the bony arch formed at the junction of the cheek bones (*malar* bones) and *temporal* bones.

FASCIA, MUSCLES AND TENDONS

ANALYSIS, DEFINITIONS AND NARRATIONS

Example Terms

ABDUCTOR POLLICIS BREVIS: (*polleo* = I am strong; *brevis* = short) a muscle which flexes the thumb. *Pollex* (thumb) was derived from *polleo* because the thumb is stronger than the other fingers.

ANCONEUS: (*ankon* = elbow) a muscle which extends the forearm.

Example Terms

AURICULARIS: (*auricula,* diminutive of *auris* = ear) the muscle which moves the external ear.

BICEPS BRACHII: (*bi* = two; *caput* = head) a muscle with two heads which flexes and supinates the forearm.

BUCCINATOR: (*buccinator* = a trumpeter) the muscle of the cheek.

CREMASTER: (*kremastos* = hanging) the muscle on which the testis is hung.

DELTOIDEUS: (*delta* = the Greek letter Δ) a triangular muscle which abducts and rotates the humerus.

DIAPHRAGMA: (*phragma* = a fence) a wall of muscle between the thoracic and abdominal cavities; used in respiration.

DIGASTRICUS: (*di* = double; *gaster* = belly) the muscle which lifts the tongue and the hyoid bone. It has two "bellies."

FASCIA: (*fascia* = a ribbon or fillet) the sheets of connective tissue which bind other tissues. (*Fascist* comes from *fasces* = a bundle of rods around an axe, symbolizing power; the bundle was tied with a *fascia.*)

FLEXOR CARPI ULNARIS: (*flectere* = to bend) a muscle which flexes the wrist.

FLEXOR DIGITORUM SUBLIMIS: (*digitus* = finger; *sublimis* = above) a muscle which flexes the second phalanges.

GASTROCNEMIUS: (*kneme* = the lower leg) the muscle of the calf of the leg; the "belly" of the leg.

GEMELLUS SUPERIOR: (*gemellus* = a twin) one of two similar muscles which rotate the thigh outwards.

GENIOGLOSSUS: (*geneion* = the chin; *glossus,* from *glossa* = tongue) the muscle which protrudes and retracts the tongue.

GLUTEUS MAXIMUS: (*gloutos* = buttock) the largest of the buttock muscles; extends, abducts and rotates the thigh outward.

Example Terms

GRACILIS: (*gracilis* = slender) a muscle which flexes and abducts the legs.

LATISSIMUS DORSI: (superlative of *latus* = broad) the broadest muscle of the back; it draws the arm backwards and downwards and rotates it inwards.

LEVATOR PALPEBRAE SUPERIORIS: (*levare* = to lift; *palpebra* = eyelid) the muscle which lifts the upper eyelid.

LIGAMENT: (*ligare* = to bind) a tough fibrous band which connects and supports.

LUMBRICALES: (*lumbricus* = an earthworm) intrinsic muscles of the hand, named for their supposed resemblance to worms.

MASSETER: (*maseter* = chewer) the muscles of mastication.

ORBICULARIS OCULI: (*orbicularis* = circular, disk-shaped) the muscle which closes the eye.

PECTINEUS: (*pecten* = a comb) a muscle which flexes the thigh and rotates it outwards. Its fibers are supposed to resemble the prongs or teeth of a comb.

PECTORALIS MAJOR: (*pectus* = thorax) the large chest muscle which draws the arm downward and forward.

PERONEUS LONGUS: (*perone* = a brooch or pin) a muscle which extends and everts the foot. The peroneus muscles are so called because they are attached to the fibula.

PIRIFORMIS: (*pirum* = a pear) a muscle, named for its shape, which rotates the thigh outwards.

POPLITEUS: (*poples* = the ham, or back of the knee) a muscle which flexes the leg. The Roman soldiers, with their short skirts or kilts, were especially vulnerable to "hamstringing" by a cut at the back of the knee.

PROCERUS: (*procerus* = stretching up) the muscle which depresses the eyebrow.

Example Terms

PRONATOR TERES: (*pronare* = to turn face downward; *teres* = smooth) a smooth muscle which turns the hand palm downwards.

PSOAS MAJOR: (*psoa* = loin muscle) a muscle which flexes and rotates the thigh outward and flexes the trunk and pelvis.

PTERYGOIDEUS: (*pteryx* = wing; *oid* = resembles) winglike muscles which move the lower jaws.

RECTUS: (*rectus* = straight) four eye muscles have this description, i.e., *r. superior oculi, r. inferior oculi, r. lateralis oculi, r. medialis oculi.*

RHOMBOIDEUS MAJOR: (*rhombos* = a lozenge) a lozenge-shaped muscle which elevates and retracts the shoulder blade.

RISORIUS: (*risor* = one who laughs) the muscle which draws the corner of the mouth outwards.

SARTORIUS: (*sartor* = a tailor) a muscle which flexes and crosses the legs. Called the "tailor's muscle" because, anciently, tailors squatted with their legs crossed.

SCALENUS: (*skalenos* = uneven) three muscles which move the neck. They form, roughly, a triangle with unequal sides.

SERRATI POSTERIORES: (*serra* = saw) muscles which move the ribs; they have notched edges.

SPHINCTER and EXTERNUS: (*sphingein* = to bind; *externus* = outside) the muscle which closes the anus.

SPLENIUS: (*splenion* = bandage) a muscle at the back of the neck which is wrapped round the other deep muscles like a bandage.

STERNOCLEIDOMASTOIDEUS: (*sternon* = breastbone; *kleis* = key; *mastos* = breast) the muscle which depresses and rotates the head. It originates in two places (sternum and clavicle) and attaches to the mastoid process of the skull.

Example Terms

SUPINATOR: (*supinare* = to turn face upward) a muscle which turns the hand palm upward.

TENDON: (*tendere* = to stretch) the elongated part of a muscle stretched to grasp and hold fast to the bone.

TENSOR VELI PALATINI: (*tensor* = puller; *veli* = veil; *palatum* = palate) the muscle which tautens the soft palate.

TERES MAJOR: (*teres* = round, smooth) a cylindrical muscle which draws the arm down and back.

CONDITIONS AND DISEASES OF MUSCULOSKELETAL SYSTEM

(Here, analyses of most of the terms given previously have been omitted. The student might use these terms as study exercises in analysis.)

ANALYSIS, DEFINITION AND NARRATIONS

Example Terms

ACHONDROPLASIA: a type of dwarfism due to premature ossification and closure of the epiphyseal lines.

BELL'S PALSY: facial paralysis due to neuritis of the facial nerve.

COXA VALGA: is the opposite of coxa vara (see next term).

COXA VARA: (*coxa* = the hip; *vara* = bent) a bending downward of the hip in which the angle of the femoral neck with the shaft is reduced below 130°.

CONGENITAL CLUBFOOT: (*talipes equinovarus*) consists of plantar flexion of the foot on the leg (*equinus*) and inversion of the foot (*varus*) and usually adduction of the forefoot.

CONGENITAL DISLOCATION OF THE HIPS: a condition in which the head of the femur lies outside the acetabulum. It may be unilateral or bilateral.

Example Terms

DISLOCATION: a separation of the bones from a joint.

DYSCHONDROPLASIA: a condition of abnormal formation of cartilage in which the ends of the long bones are distorted.

DYSTROPHIA MYOTONIA CONGENITA: (Thomson's disease) an hereditary condition characterized by muscle spasm when attempting to relax grasp.

FIBROSITIS: inflammation of fascia and muscle sheaths.

FRACTURES: (*fractura* = a break) may be simple, compound, incomplete, comminuted, impacted, compressive, sprain-fracture, spontaneous, pathological.

GONOCOCCAL ARTHRITIS: inflammation of joints due to gonococcus microorganism.

GOUT: (*podagra*) deposits of uric acid crystals in the joints, especially of the feet.

HYPERTROPHIC ARTHRITIS: a degenerative disease of the joints of unknown cause, characterized by the irregular overgrowth of new bone.

KYPHOSIS: hump-back (a type of curvature of spine).

LEGG-CALVÉ-PERTHES' DISEASE: osteochondritis of the head of the femur.

LORDOSIS: swayback.

MYASTHENIA GRAVIS: (*gravis* = heavy) rapid fatigue of the muscles without pain.

MYOSITIS: inflammation of muscle.

OSTEITIS FIBROSA CYSTICA: (von Recklinghausen's disease) a bony manifestation of hyperparathyroidism.

OSTEITIS DEFORMANS: (Paget's disease) a generalized disease of the bones in adults, characterized by enlargement and distortion.

Example Terms

OSTEOCHONDRITIS: a destructive inflammation of bone and cartilage.

OSTEOCHONDRITIS DISSECANS: development of a loose body in a joint. The loose body is cartilage with a layer of bone beneath.

OSTEOGENESIS IMPERFECTA: a condition (usually prepubertal) in which the bones are brittle and fracture easily.

OSTEOMALACIA: "adult rickets," with softening of bone.

PROGRESSIVE MUSCULAR ATROPHY: a condition in which the muscles waste progressively.

PROGRESSIVE MUSCULAR DYSTROPHY: progressive muscular impairment with no discoverable lesion of spinal cord.

RHEUMATIC FEVER: An acute febrile polyarthritis, often with associated heart involvement.

RHEUMATOID ARTHRITIS: (*rheuma* = flux; *oid* = resembling) resembling rheumatism; a chronic disease of the joints in which the bone is atrophied and the synovial membrane hypertrophied.

RICKETS: a deficiency disease of early childhood characterized by failure of bone tissue to calcify.

SCOLIOSIS: an abnormal lateral curvature of the spine.

SLIPPED EPIPHYSIS: the separation of epiphysis from diaphysis occurring in young children, caused by excessive trauma.

SPINA BIFIDA: (*bifidus* = split in two) a failure of the spinal arches to close, permitting protrusion of the membranes (meningocele).

SPONDYLOLISTHESIS: (*spondylos* = vertebra; *olisthesis* = a slipping) the forward displacement of one vertebra on another.

SYPHILITIC ARTHRITIS: inflammation of joints occurring in the secondary stage of syphilis.

Example Terms

TENOSYNOVITIS: inflammation of a tendon sheath.

TORTICOLLIS: (*tortus* = twisted; *collum* = neck) wryneck.

TUBERCULOUS ARTHRITIS: inflammation due to *Mycobacterium tuberculosis,* involving joints of the hip and spine, usually in children and young adults.

RESPIRATORY SYSTEM

RESPIRATION: (*re* = again; *spirare* = to breathe). It implies the function of inspiration and expiration.

ANATOMICAL PARTS

ANALYSIS, DEFINITIONS AND NARRATIONS

Example Terms

ALVEOLUS: (*alveolus* = a small space) a small hollow space in the lung; the air sac.

BRONCHIOLE: a diminutive of bronchus. A little windpipe or the terminals of air conduction.

BRONCHUS: (*bronchos* = windpipe; perhaps from *brechein* = to moisten) a primary extension of the trachea. The earlier anatomists believed that liquids were carried by the bronchus and solid food by the esophagus.

GLOTTIS: (*glottis* = the reed of a wind instrument). In earlier times it meant the mouthpiece of a flute. It is a space between the vocal cords, which, aided by larynx, tongue, lips and teeth, helps to produce sound and form words.

LARYNX: (*larynx* = upper part of windpipe) the organ of the voice.

LUNG: (*lungre* = quickly or lightly) the organ of respiration. The lungs are light of weight and can float on water. This may account for the fact that the lay term for lungs is "lights."

NARES: (*naris* = nostril; pl. is *nares*) external openings of nasal cavities.

Example Terms

PLEURA: (*pleura* = rib, or the side of an animal) the serous membrane enveloping the lung.

SEPTUM: (*saeptum* = fence) a dividing wall between the nasal cavities (not to be confused with *septem,* meaning "seven").

SINUS: (*sinuare* = swell out in a curve) a pocket. In this category, the sinuses are air cavities in one of the cranial bones communicating with the nose and more correctly referred to as the paranasal sinuses.

TRACHEA: (*tracheia* = rough) the windpipe, called by the ancients *arteria tracheia.* They thought the arteries contained air, hence the term *artery,* which means "air vessel." The windpipe was the "rough artery," from its corrugations.

TURBINATES: (*turbo* = whirl-shaped) curled flakes of bone in nasal cavity. The meaning of whirl as applied here is not particularly apt, since these bones shape to a mere curve.

CONDITIONS AND DISEASES OF RESPIRATORY SYSTEM

ANALYSIS, DEFINITIONS AND NARRATIONS

(Analysis of terms given previously is not repeated)

Example Terms

ACUTE RHINITIS: (*rhis, rhin* = nose) infection of the mucosa of the nasal passages.

ASTHMA: (*asthma* = a panting) a disease involving the bronchus, characterized by paroxysmal attacks of dyspnea. It is usually due to an allergy.

ATELECTASIS: (*atel* = imperfect; *ectasis* = dilatation) a condition in which the lung tissue is collapsed.

BRONCHIECTASIS: a dilatation of the bronchi.

BRONCHOPNEUMONIA: inflammation of the lungs which usually begins in the terminal bronchioles.

Example Terms

CYSTIC FIBROSIS OF LUNG: see under cystic fibrosis of digestive system.

EDEMA OF THE LARYNX: (*oidema* = a swelling) a swelling of the larynx.

EMPHYSEMA: a condition in which the lung or a part of it is abnormally distended with air.

EPISTAXIS: (*epistazein* = to trickle drop by drop) a nosebleed, may be due to ulceration of the nasal septum, trauma or hypertension.

LOBAR PNEUMONIA: inflammation of the lobes of the lung, usually caused by pneumococcus.

PNEUMOTHORAX: an accumulation of air in the pleural cavity.

STENOSIS OF TRACHEA AND BRONCHI: (*stenos* = narrow) a partial closure of the organs involved.

TRACHEO-ESOPHAGEAL FISTULA: (*fistula* = a tube) an opening between the trachea and esophagus.

CARDIOVASCULAR SYSTEM

(Specialist in this field is usually the Cardiologist)

CARDIOVASCULAR: (*cardia* = heart; *vasculum*, a diminutive of *vas* = vessel, or vase) means pertaining to the heart and blood vessels.

ANATOMICAL PARTS

ANALYSIS, DEFINITIONS AND NARRATIONS

Example Terms

ARTERY: (*aer* = air; *terein* = to keep) a vessel which carries blood from the heart to the tissues of the body. The ancients thought that arteries were pipes to carry or contain air. This belief was due to their observation that after death most of the blood collected in the veins, leaving the arteries empty.

Example Terms

CAPILLARIES: (*capilli* = hair of head; hence *capillaris* = anything hairlike) threadlike tubes; small blood vessels.

INTERSTITIAL TISSUE: (*sistere* = to stand) tissue which stands at intervals in an organ or tissue.

JUGULAR VEIN: (*jugulum* = throat; from *jugum* = yoke) a vein collecting blood from the head and neck to return it to the heart. The jugular vein was once regarded as the sacrificial vein.

MITRAL VALVE: (*mitra* = mitre, cap) the bicuspid valve of the heart. The valve cusps have something of the appearance of a bishop's headdress, but not much.

SAPHENOUS VEINS: (*saphenes* = clear, manifest) veins of the lower limb, situated just below the surface of the skin.

TRICUSPID VALVE: (*cuspis* = a point) a valve of the heart having three leaflets.

VEIN: (*vena* = vein) a vessel which carries blood from the tissues back to the heart. Ancient writers failed to distinguish between arteries and veins. It was thought by some that veins arose in the liver and arteries in the heart. In later years, after circulation had been fully described and understood, a distinction was made between arteries and veins.

VENTRICLE: (*venter* = the belly; plus the diminutive *culus* = a little belly, hence any small cavity) one of the chambers of the heart.

CONDITIONS AND DISEASES OF CARDIOVASCULAR SYSTEM

ANALYSIS, DEFINITIONS AND NARRATIONS

Example Terms

ARTERIOSCLEROSIS: a hardening and thickening of the artery walls with loss of elasticity, formation of fibrous tissue and possibly calcification, causing cardiac hypertrophy and high blood pressure.

Example Terms

BACTERIAL ENDOCARDITIS: inflammation around the heart valves due to the presence of microorganisms.

CARDIAC DILATATION: a dilatation of the heart muscle.

CARDIAC HYPERTROPHY: a condition in which a ventricle enlarges as the result of some abnormal condition.

CONGENITAL PULMONARY STENOSIS: (*pulmo* = lung) a child born with a partial closing of the pulmonary artery.

CORONARY SCLEROSIS: a disease in which the coronary arteries thicken, lose elasticity and possibly calcify, thus decreasing their diameter and depriving the heart of an adequate blood supply.

DEXTROCARDIA: placement of the heart on the right side in the thoracic cavity.

HEMOPERICARDIUM: blood in the pericardial sac.

HYDROPERICARDIUM: abnormal increase in fluid in the pericardial sac.

HYPERTENSIVE HEART: a condition in which the heart has to work against increased peripheral resistance due to high blood pressure in the arteries.

PERICARDITIS: inflammation of the pericardium.

PHLEBITIS: an inflammation of the veins generally caused by an inflammatory, suppurative process elsewhere in the body. (See prefix *phlebo*.)

RAYNAUD'S DISEASE: a disturbance in the vasomotor mechanism of the artery in which spasm of the arteries causes anemia in the part of the body supplied by them, usually fingers and toes.

RHEUMATIC ENDOCARDITIS: a disease in which the heart valves show many small firm vegetations. This condition is the most frequent complication of rheumatic fever.

Example Terms

THROMBOANGIITIS OBLITERANS: (Buerger's disease) involves the larger arteries of the body, especially of the leg, and often results in gangrene. The vessels become occluded by firm thrombi. The cause is unknown.

VARICOSE VEINS: (*varix* = enlarged and tortuous vein). They are usually due to increased intravenous pressure, occasionally to hereditary weakness of the vein wall. The important *varices* (pl. of *varix*) include *hemorrhoids,* varix of the esophagus, *varicose veins of the legs,* and *varicocele* (varicosity of the spermatic veins).

HEMIC AND LYMPHATIC SYSTEM

(Specialist in this field is the Hematologist)

HEMIC: (*haima* = blood) pertaining to the blood.

LYMPHATIC: (*lympha* = clear water) pertaining to the tissue fluids.

ANATOMICAL PARTS

ANALYSIS, DEFINITIONS AND NARRATIONS

Example Terms

ERYTHROBLAST: (*blastos* = germ) a precursor of erythrocyte; an immature red cell.

ERYTHROCYTE: (*erythros* = red; *kytos* = cell) a red blood cell.

ERYTHROPOIETIC TISSUE: (*erythros* = red; *poiesis* = making) tissue in which red blood cells are produced.

LYMPH NODES: (*nodus* = a knot) small oval masses of lymphatic tissue occurring along the course of lymph glands. They act as filters of impurities.

MARROW: (from *mearh,* an Anglo-Saxon term; the Latin term is *medulla*). It is a meshwork of connective tissue which fills the bones.

Example Terms

MYELOID TISSUE: (*myelos* = marrow; *oid* = resemblance) tissue resembling bone marrow.

PLASMA: (anything molded) the fluid part of blood in which corpuscles are suspended.

SPLEEN: prefix is *splen* or *lien*. Its function is to disintegrate the red blood cells and free the hemoglobin.

RETICULOENDOTHELIAL SYSTEM: (*rete* = net; *culum* = small; *endo* = within; *thele* = nipple). This system is a network concerned in blood cell formation, the storage of fat, and destruction of infection within the cells. It is the network of cells in the liver, spleen, bone marrow and hemolymph nodes.

CONDITIONS AND DISEASES OF HEMIC AND LYMPHATIC SYSTEM

ANALYSIS, DEFINITIONS AND NARRATIONS

Example Terms

ANEMIA: a decrease in the number of circulating red blood cells.

HEMOPHILIA: an inherited disease in which the blood clots so slowly that the slightest injury causes severe bleeding.

HYPERPLASIA OF THE THYMUS: an increase in the number of cells in the thymus.

LEUKEMIA: a disease characterized by marked increase in the number of white cells for an allotted area of tissue.

LEUKOCYTOSIS: an abnormal increase in the number of white blood cells, present in almost every sort of infection.

LEUKOPENIA: (*penia* = poverty) a decrease in the number of white blood cells.

LYMPHADENITIS: acute or chronic inflammation of the lymph nodes, characterized by swelling and tenderness.

POLYCYTHEMIA: an increase in the number of circulating red blood cells.

Example Terms

PURPURA: (*purpura* = purple) a term used for a variety of hemorrhagic states in which spontaneous bleeding occurs beneath the skin.

DIGESTIVE SYSTEM

(Specialist in this field is the Gastroenterologist)

DIGESTIVE: (*digestio* = breakup, from *dis* = apart and *gerere* = to carry) pertaining to the assimilation of food by a process of breaking up.

ALIMENTARY TRACT: (*alimentum* = nourishment, from *alere* = to nourish) the digestive tract; sometimes called the gastrointestinal tract.

ANATOMICAL PARTS

ANALYSIS, DEFINITIONS AND NARRATIONS

Example Terms

ACINAR TISSUE: (*acinum* = a grape). Small saclike lobules or dilatations like grapes.

ADENOID: (*aden* = gland; *oid* = resemblance) hypertrophied lymph tissue in the nasopharynx; the name refers to a supposed resemblance in appearance to a gland.

ALVEOLUS: diminutive of *alveus,* meaning any hollowed-out structure. Plural is *alveoli.* The tooth socket is an example.

AMPULLA: (*ampulla* = flask or jug) discovered by Abraham Vater (1684-1751), German anatomist. The ampulla of Vater is the expanded portion at the entrance of the common bile duct and the pancreatic duct into the duodenum.

ANUS: (*anus* = a ring; possibly Sanskrit *as* = to sit) the terminal orifice of the alimentary canal. There is some confusion as to the origin of this term. It was first spoken of as the opening of the intestines, and is now called the outlet.

APPENDIX: (*pendere* = to hang) a pendulum; a small pouch pendant from the cecum. Sometimes called the vermiform (*vermis* = a worm) appendix.

Example Terms

BILE: (*bilis* = bile) the golden-brown or greenish-yellow substance secreted by the liver.

BRANCHIAL VESTIGES: (*branchion* = gill of fishes or a cleft; *vestigium* = a footprint or trace mark, a remnant or degenerative part). Before birth, there is an outstanding peculiarity in the walls of the pharynx; they are not of uniform thickness throughout, but are covered with thin places alternating with thick places. The thin places are called branchial grooves; the thick places are called branchial arches. The branchial vestiges, then, are the remnants of this prenatal development. The branchial arches disappear in a baby except as they are represented in the jaws; the branchial grooves are almost obliterated except the part which becomes the external auditory canal.

CECUM: (*caecus* = blind) the blind gut or the blind end of the large intestine. The ileum, appendix and colon open into it.

COLON: (*kolon* = food) the large intestine, divided into cecum, ascending colon, transverse colon, descending colon, sigmoid and rectum.

DUCT: (*ducere* = to lead) a tube or channel, especially one for conveying the secretion of a gland.

DUODENUM: (*duodeni* = twelve). By measurement, this part of the intestine was found to be twelve fingerbreadths in length; thus, its name.

ESOPHAGUS: (*oesophagus* = gullet). The gullet; the tube which carries food between pharynx and stomach.

GLAND: (*glandula* = a gland; diminutive of *glans* = an acorn) an organ which secretes something essential to the system or excretes waste. The name is assumed to come from a supposed similarity to an acorn.

ILEUM: (*ilis* = soft; *ileum* = abdomen). The lower portion of the small intestine, terminating in the cecum. "It was found to be the colicky part of the gut, while the jejunum was

Example Terms

always found to be the empty gut." *Ilium,* the bone, and *ileum,* a part of the intestine, may originate from the same word, probably because of their apparent proximity.

INTESTINE: (*intestinus* = internal; from *intus* = within) the part of the alimentary canal from the pylorus to the anus.

JEJUNUM: (*jejunus* = hungry or fasting) the portion of the small intestine which follows the duodenum. Named by the ancients because at death it was always found to be empty.

LIVER: (Anglo-Saxon *lifer* = liver) the largest gland in the body, with many functions, including the secretion of bile, the production and destruction of blood capsules, the production and storage of glycogen, etc. Various other old spellings are livre, lyvre, lyvour, lyffere, lywer, liffre, luffer and livour. An ancient notion was that the liver was the seat of love and of violent passion generally. Dryden wrote, "When Love's unerring Dart transfixt his liver and inflam'd his Heart." A white liver was spoken of as characterizing a coward. Also sometimes the word liver has been used to mean temperament, such as in "John Bull will solumly and dully sit down to his pipe's bowl with a fellow of the same liver."

MECKEL'S DIVERTICULUM: (*divertere* = to turn aside; plus the diminutive *culum.* Meckel = Johann Friedrich Meckel, the Younger, a German anatomist.) A little turn-aside, a bypath or branch road. In this instance, a pouch off the ileum, discovered by Meckel.

MESENTERY: (*meson* = middle; *enteron* = bowel) middle portion between intestines; the membranous structure spreading itself like a sheet and connecting the different portions of intestine together as well as attaching itself to the posterior abdominal wall to stabilize positions of organs.

PALATE: (*palatum* = the roof of the mouth, which was formerly called the diaphragm of the mouth, or *diaphragma oris*). The origin of the term is uncertain. Its origin has been associated with:

Example Terms

   (1) *pascere* = to feed; or

   (2) *palere* = to hedge in (because it is hedged in by teeth) ; or

   (3) *balatus* = bleating (this version refers to the Palatine Hill in Rome, a name which is said to come from *balatus* and was so called because of the bleating flocks of sheep which grazed there. The palate would be the bleating organ associated with the voice). (Campbell's *Language of Medicine*)

PANCREAS: (*pan* = all; *kreas* = flesh). An organ which appears to be all flesh, the sweetbread. Its chief secretion, insulin, helps to control carbohydrate distribution.

PAROTID GLAND: (*para* = beside; *oto* = ear) the gland beside the ear; actually, just in front of the ear.

PERICHOLECYSTIC TISSUE: (*peri* = around; *chole* = bile; *kystis* = saclike or bladder) tissue around the bile bladder or gall bladder.

PHARYNX: (*pharynx* = throat) the pouch at the back of the nose, mouth and larynx.

PYLORUS: (*pyle* = gate; *ouros* = a guard) gate-keeper. It is the muscular ring part which guards the outlet of the stomach.

RECTUM : (*rectus* = straight) so named by Galen because he found it straight in lower animals; in man it does not warrant this name. In ancient times Hippocrates referred to the rectum as *archos* = chief or first.

SALIVARY GLANDS: (*saliva* = the juices of the mouth) glands which produce tasteless alkaline mixture of secreta to moisten food.

SEROSA: (*serum*) the fluid part of whey, so called by the Latins because it resembled the watery part of curdled milk. It acts as a lubricant to membranous linings. A membrane producing serum.

Example Terms

SIGMOID COLON: (*sigma* = the Greek letter "s") a structure which is S-shaped. The final form of sigma is written with a single curve resembling "C", and this shape is appropriate to the bowel curve we call sigmoid.

STOMACH: (*stomachos* = a mouth, an opening, from *stoma*) the most dilated part of the alimentary canal, where food is digested prior to its delivery to the tissues. Originally this name was applied to the esophagus, with the idea that the gullet was the mouth of the stomach. The Greek *stomachos* became the Latin *stomachus,* mouth of the ventriculus, while the esophagus became the *via stomachi,* or the road to the stomach.

TONGUE: (Anglo-Saxon *tunga*) the movable muscular organ in the mouth, an agent in tasting, chewing, swallowing and speech. The word tongue, from a teutonic root, may be an imitation of the French word *langue*. The old Latin form was *dingua,* which later developed into *lingua*. The Greek is *glossa*.

TONSIL: (*tonsilla* = a pole stuck in the ground and used as a mooring post). The reason for applying this term is not known. Could it be because the tonsils are a mooring for bacteria, bound there until the phagocytes have fought off their virulence?

UVULA: (*uva* = a grape cluster; *ula* = diminutive suffix) a little grape cluster, so called because of the resemblance. It is a small conical appendage hanging from the free edge of the soft palate.

CONDITIONS AND DISEASES OF DIGESTIVE SYSTEM

ANALYSIS, DEFINITIONS AND NARRATIONS

Example Terms

ACUTE CATARRHAL JAUNDICE: believed to be due to injury to the liver cells.

ACUTE GASTRITIS: acute inflammation of the stomach.

Example Terms

ACUTE YELLOW ATROPHY: a disease of unknown cause, but is a sequel of many infectious diseases.

ATROPHY OF THE LIVER: a decrease in size and function of the liver.

ATROPHY OF THE TONGUE: a decrease in size and function of the tongue; may occur in pernicious anemia and other diseases.

BILIARY CALCULI: stones in the bile passages.

CHOLANGITIS: inflammation of the bile ducts.

CHOLECYSTITIS: an inflammation of the gall bladder, which may be acute, subacute or chronic.

CHOLELITHIASIS: stones in the bile passages.

CIRRHOSIS OF THE LIVER: (*kirros* = tawny yellow) is a slowly progressive chronic degeneration and reparative process, believed to be inflammatory in origin.

COLITIS: inflammation of the colon.

CONGESTION OF THE LIVER: if chronic and passive, is due to heart failure and is simply a backing up of blood in the liver.

CYSTIC FIBROSIS or MUCOVISCIDOSIS: Generally considered an abnormality of the secreting glands such as those that manufacture mucus and sweat. It can become generalized, affecting all glands that secrete fluid into the body cavities or from the skin. More noticeably the pancreas and lungs are involved. The mucus is thick and sticky and the sweat glands have a high concentration of salt. When the lungs are affected the bronchi and trachea are filled with thick mucus and the passageways are blocked. The result may be persistent cough, wheezing, dyspnea and emphysema. When the pancreas is affected there is marked disturbance of the bowel, and glandular cells lining other organs affect the stomach juices, saliva, bile and other structures. Patients are likely to perspire profusely and loss of large amounts of salt may result in heat exhaustion.

Example Terms

DENTAL CARIES: (*caries* = dry rot) decalcification of the dental enamel leading to dental decay.

DIVERTICULUM OF THE ESOPHAGUS: an outpocketing, congenital or acquired.

ENTERITIS: inflammation of the intestine.

GASTROPTOSIS: a falling of the stomach.

HEPATITIS: inflammation of the liver. Infection may enter the liver at many points, e.g., portal vein, hepatic artery, bile ducts.

IMPERFORATE ANUS: a rare congenital condition in which the rectum ends as a blind pouch.

INFARCTION OF INTESTINE: (*infarcire* = to stuff, i.e., to fill up) necrosis of the intestine due to lack of blood supply.

LEUKOPLAKIA: (*plax*= a plaque or flake) tough white spots on the tongue or elsewhere in the mouth; may be due to chronic irritation.

MUMPS: (*mump* = a grimace) a virus infection of the parotid gland. Another word for mumps is infectious parotitis.

PANCREATITIS: inflammation of the pancreas.

PEPTIC ULCER: may occur in the stomach mucosa (gastric ulcer) or in the first part of the duodenum (duodenal ulcer) and may be in one of three stages, viz., hemorrhagic erosion, acute ulcer or chronic ulcer.

PERITONSILLAR ABSCESS: accumulation of pus around the tonsils.

PYORRHEA ALVEOLARIS: inflammation of the gums and the roots of the teeth leading to the formation of pus.

STENOSIS OF THE ESOPHAGUS: partial closure which may be congenital or caused by pressure from a growth.

VINCENT'S ANGINA: ulcers in the mouth, due to an infection with Vincent's organism.

UROGENITAL SYSTEM

UROGENITAL SYSTEM: (*ouron* = urine; *genere* = to produce) the combined systems of the urinary tract and organs of reproduction.

ANATOMICAL PARTS OF
URINARY SYSTEM

(Specialist practicing in this field is the Urologist)

ANALYSIS, DEFINITIONS AND NARRATIONS

Example Terms

GLOMERULI: pl. of *glomerulus* (*glomus* = a ball; *ulus* = a diminutive) little coils of blood vessels projecting into the expanded end of the urine-bearing tubules of the kidney.

HILUS: (*hilum* = a small thing; a trifle) point at which the kidney vessels enter and leave the organ. Hilus is corruption of *hilum*. *Hilum* was used by the Romans for the little spot on a seed which marked its point of attachment; especially noticeable on the bean. The Romans would say a thing was *ne hilum*, that is, "not worth a hilum," whereas the English say "not worth a bean." The word *nihil*, meaning nothing, comes from *ne hilum*. A further contraction is the word *nil*.

KIDNEY: (Middle English *kidenei*) a glandular organ which secretes and excretes urine. The origin of the name is not known although some think it may be a corruption of the Icelandic word for womb, which is *kid*.

PARENCHYMA: (*para* = beside; *en* = in; *chymos* = juice or infusion). In the kidney, the parenchyma are the secreting elements.

RENAL CALICES: pl. of calix (*ren* = kidney; *calix* = a cup) cuplike recesses of the kidney pelvis which receive the urine.

RENAL PELVIS: (*ren* = kidney; *pelvis* = tub, trough or basin) the basin or cavity of the kidney which is drained by the ureter.

Example Terms

TRIGONE: (*tri* = three; *gonia* = angle) a triangular area of the interior of the bladder between the opening of the ureters and mouth of urethra.

URACHUS: (*ouron* = urine; *echein* = to hold) hold or pouch for urine in the fetus. It is a remnant of the allantoic canal (*allas* = sausage), the part of the fetus where urine is stored. It connects with the bladder before birth. If the allantoic canal persists after birth, it is called a "patent urachus" (*patent* = open).

URETER: (*ouron* = urine) the tube which carries urine from kidney to bladder.

URETEROVESICAL: (*vesica* = blister or bladder). This term refers to ureter and urinary bladder. The urinary bladder is the reservoir for urine.

URETHRA: (*ourein* = to make water; to urinate) a canal carrying urine from the urinary bladder to the surface. The organ of urination.

VERUMONTANUM: (*veru* = skewer or spit for roasting; *montanus* = mountainous). A ridge or crest of the urethra. It has other names, one being the "caput gallinaginis," meaning woodcock's head.

MALE GENITAL ORGANS

(Except for endocrine diseases, the specialist in this field is the Urologist)

ANALYSIS, DEFINITIONS AND NARRATIONS

Example Terms

CORPORA CAVERNOSA: (*corpus* = body; *cavernosus* = containing caverns or hollows). Cavernous bodies or spongy bodies; the two erectile columns of the penis of the male or clitoris of the female.

Example Terms

EPIDIDYMIS: (*epi* = upon; *didymos* = twin). Didymos was a botanical term meaning twin and later used to indicate the testicles since there are two. The epididymis is the duct of the testicle.

PENIS: (*penis* or *glans penis;* also *penis* = a tail) the male sexual organ.

PREPUCE: (*praeputium* = foreskin) the foreskin of the penis.

PROSTATE GLAND: (*pro* = before; *histemi* = to stand) the gland in front of the bladder in the male. Its secretion stimulates the motility of the spermatozoa. In Greece, a *prostates* was a guard who stood in front of a place or an object as its protector.

SCROTUM: (*scrotum* = hide, or *scrotea* = leather jacket). Scrotum, as used in medicine, seems to be a corruptive usage. It is the pouch containing the testicles and their accessory parts.

SEMINAL VESICLES: (*semen* = seed; from *serere* = to sow; *vesicula* = a little bladder or bag) the sacs containing the spermatozoa; the seed bag.

SPERMATOZOA: (*sperma* = seed; *zoon* = a living thing) the plural of spermatozoon, meaning the male seed or germ.

TESTIS or TESTICLE: (*testum* = a pot, or *testis* = a witness). It is a curious fact that the Latin word for testicle is the same as the Latin word for witness. For the purpose of interest, the narrations on derivations might be as follows:

The *testum* was an earthen pot in which tests were made by chemists. From this meaning came our word "test tube." Another version is that the word *testa* meant a shell. Shells were used in voting. This is thought to have been the origin of the terms "testify" and "testament." Thus, *testis* was one who voted. Having voted, one is of age or has come to manhood, and manhood indicates virility.

Example Terms

The testis is an egg-shaped gland in the scrotum which produces spermatozoa, the male germ or seed causing reproduction or pregnancy.

TUNICA VAGINALIS: (*tunica* = shirt; *vagina* = a sheath). This term is used to describe the sheathlike, serous covering of the testis. It is formed by a portion of the peritoneum, which descends with the testicle and later forms a pouch which encloses the testicles.

VAS DEFERENS: (*vas* = vessel or vase; *de* = away; *ferre* = to carry) the duct which carries the excretions away from the testicles.

CONDITIONS AND DISEASES OF THE URINARY AND MALE GENITAL SYSTEMS

ANALYSIS, DEFINITIONS AND NARRATIONS

Example Terms

BALANITIS: (*balanos* = an acorn) inflammation of the glans penis.

BENIGN PROSTATIC HYPERTROPHY: a tumor-like enlargement of the prostate.

CHANCRE: a primary ulcerative lesion of syphilis, usually on the glans penis.

CRYPTORCHISM: a congenital condition in which one or both testes fail to descend into the scrotum.

CYSTITIS: an inflammation of the urinary bladder, most frequently caused by stagnant urine.

EPIDIDYMITIS: an inflammation of the epididymis due to microorganisms.

EXSTROPHY OF THE BLADDER: a congenital absence of its anterior and of the abdominal wall in front of it, the posterior wall of the bladder being exposed.

Example Terms

GLOMERULAR NEPHRITIS, NONSUPPURATIVE: (Bright's disease) inflammation of the glomeruli.

HORSESHOE KIDNEY: an anomaly due to the fusion of the lower poles of the kidney, giving it a horseshoe shape.

HYDROCELE: an accumulation of fluid in the *tunica vaginalis*.

HYDRONEPHROSIS: a dilatation of the kidney pelvis due to pressure from the excess fluid present.

HYPERTROPHY OF THE KIDNEY: results in an abnormally large organ.

ORCHITIS: inflammation of the testes.

PHIMOSIS: (*phimos* = a muzzle) a narrowing of the prepuce so that it cannot be retracted over the glans penis. It may be congenital or inflammatory in origin.

POLYCYSTIC KIDNEYS: are filled with cysts which enlarge the kidney and compress the renal tissue.

PROSTATITIS: inflammation of the prostate.

PYELITIS: a bacterial inflammation of the kidney pelvis.

PYELONEPHRITIS: infection of the kidney and kidney pelvis as a result of some obstruction to the flow of urine.

SPERMATOCELE: a cystic dilatation of the epididymis.

SUPPURATIVE NEPHRITIS: is characterized by the presence of abscesses and bacteria.

URETERAL STRICTURE: (*strictura* = a binding) generally occurs at the origin of the ureter in the kidney pelvis or just before its entrance into the bladder.

URETHRAL STRICTURE: may occur and block the outflow of urine with resulting infection and hydronephrosis.

URINARY CALCULI: stones of various sizes in the urinary tract.

FEMALE GENITAL ORGANS

(*Note:* Except during pregnancy, the specialist practicing in this field is the Gynecologist. The Obstetrician is the specialist practicing in this field during pregnancy and through delivery of the fetus.)

ANATOMICAL PARTS

ANALYSIS, DEFINITIONS AND NARRATIONS

Example Terms

CERVIX UTERI: (*cervix* = neck; *uteri* = of the womb or uterus) the neck of the uterus.

CLITORIS: the female homologue of the penis.

CORPUS LUTEUM: (*corpus* = body; *luteum* = yellow) a yellow body which forms in the Graafian follicle after discharge of the ovum. If the ovum has been impregnated, the corpus luteum grows and lasts for several months.

GRAAFIAN FOLLICLE: (*Graafian* = from Dr. Regnier de Graaf, a Dutch anatomist; *follicle* = a little bag) the small sac in the ovary which contains the ovum or egg.

HYMEN: (*hymen* = membrane) a fold of mucous membrane partially occluding the vagina. The name originally referred to any membrane. The Greek god of marriage was Hymen, and eventually the name was restricted to the vaginal membrane, the "maidenhead."

LABIA MAJORA and LABIA MINORA: (*labium* = lip, also curved edge of a vessel) lips of the vulva. The *labia majora* are the hairy folds of skin on either side of the vulva. The *labia minora* are the folds of mucous membrane within the labia majora.

OVARY: (*ovarium* = an egg receptacle) a gland in which eggs are produced. The early Romans called the slave who had charge of the chickens and gathered the eggs, *ovarius*. The ovary was at one time called *testis muliebris* = the woman's testicle.

Example Terms

OVIDUCT: (*ovum* = egg; *ducere* = to lead) the tube which passes from the uterus to the ovary, commonly called the Fallopian tube, named after Gabriele Fallopio (1523-1562), an Italian anatomist.

PARA-, ENDO- and MYOMETRIUM: (*para* = beside; *endo* = within; *myo* = muscle; *metra* = covering of uterus). *Parametrium* is the outside covering of the uterus; *endometrium*, the inside lining and *myometrium* is the muscle structure.

UTERUS: the womb. At first the Romans used uterus only to indicate pregnant womb, but eventually it was applied to the organ without qualification.

VAGINA: (*vagina* = a sheath) a canal extending from the opening of the vulva to the mouth of the uterus.

VULVA: (*vulva* from *volvere* = to turn or wrap round) the labia and the skin covering the opening of the vagina. The name was first applied to the uterus because it wrapped around or enclosed the embryo. Later it referred to the uterine outlet, the vagina, but is now restricted to mean the extreme end of the outlet.

FETAL STRUCTURES

ANALYSIS, DEFINITIONS AND NARRATIONS

Example Terms

AMNION: (*amnion* = bowl for sacrificial blood, from *amnos* = a lamb) the membrane enclosing the fetus. How the word *amnion* came to be applied in its present sense is not known.

CHORION: (*chorion* = membrane, afterbirth) the outer membrane covering the fetal structure.

FETUS: the unborn offspring. The developing child in the uterus up to the third month is usually called an embryo. After that time, but before birth, it is called a fetus; sometimes spelled f-o-e-t-u-s.[1]

---

[1] General trend is to use anglicized spelling.

Example Terms

PLACENTA: (*placenta* = a round flat cake) a round flat organ within the uterus during pregnancy connecting mother and child by means of the umbilical cord and providing nourishment for the fetus.

SYNCYTIUM: (*syn* = together; *kytos* = cell) the outer wall of the placenta, which is a mass of epithelial cells; thus, cells together.

UMBILICAL CORD: (*umbilicus* = navel). See under regions. The cord which extends from the placenta to the fetus.

CONDITIONS AND DISEASES OF THE FEMALE GENITAL SYSTEM

ANALYSIS, DEFINITIONS AND NARRATIONS

Example Terms

ABLATIO PLACENTAE: (*ab* = away from; *latio* = carrying) premature separation of the placenta.

ABORTION: (*ab* = away from; *oriri* = to be born) spontaneous or induced delivery of the baby before it is viable.

AMENORRHEA: absence or cessation of menstruation.

DYSMENORRHEA: painful menstruation.

ECTOPIC PREGNANCY: (*gnasci* = to be born) a condition in which the fertilized ovum is implanted and develops outside the uterine cavity.

KRAUROSIS: (*krauros* = brittle or dry) a postmenopausal condition of the vulva in which there is atrophy, sclerosis and narrowing of the vaginal entrance.

LEUKOPLAKIA: a condition in which the skin of the vulva becomes parchment-like, with ulcerating points and of a white or bluish-white color.

MENOPAUSE: natural cessation of menstruation. (Natural onset is *menarche*.)

Example Terms

MENORRHAGIA: excessive menstruation.

METRORRHAGIA: abnormal uterine bleeding during the inter-menstrual period.

MULTIPARA: a woman who has had two or more pregnancies. In "para," the "p" is used to symbolize the number of pregnancies, the "a" the number of abortions, and the "ra" the number of children remaining alive. Thus multipara 2-0-3 = two pregnancies, no abortions, and 3 children (including, obviously, twins).

NULLIPARA: (*parere* = to bear) a woman who has never given birth to a child.

PLACENTA PREVIA: a condition in which the placenta develops in the region of the cervical os and complicates delivery of a child by preceding its birth.

POSTPARTUM HEMORRHAGE: Hemorrhage following delivery of a child.

PRECIPITATE LABOR: the separation and expulsion of the child and placenta occur before the usual retraction of the uterus can take place.

PRESENTATION[1] of the fetus at birth may be any of the following:

A. *Longitudinal Presentations*

  1. *Cephalic* (Head)

    a. *Occipital* (Vertex)

      (1) Left occipitoanterior — L.O.A.
      (2) Right occipitoanterior — R.O.A.
      (3) Left occipitoposterior — L.O.P.
      (4) Right occipitoposterior — R.O.P.

    b. *Sincipital* (Brow)

      (1) Left sincipitoanterior — L. Sin. A.
      (2) Right sincipitoanterior — R. Sin. A.

---

[1] Presentation: part of fetus presented at the cervix uteri.

(3) Left sincipitoposterior — L. Sin. P.

(4) Right sincipitoposterior — R. Sin. P.

c. *Mental* (Face)

(1) Left mentoanterior — L.M.A.

(2) Right mentoanterior — R.M.A.

(3) Left mentoposterior — L.M.P.

(4) Right mentoposterior — R.M.P.

2. *Pelvic* (Breech — Sacral)

(1) Left sacroanterior — L.S.A.

(2) Right sacroanterior — R.S.A.

(3) Left sacroposterior — L.S.P.

(4) Right sacroposterior — R.S.P.

B. *Transverse Presentations*

1. *Scapular* (Shoulder)

a. Left scapuloanterior — L. Sc. A.

b. Right scapuloanterior — R. Sc. A.

c. Left scapuloposterior — L. Sc. P.

d. Right scapuloposterior — R. Sc. P.

PRIMIPARA: a woman who is having her first baby.

PRURITUS OF THE VULVA: excessive itching of the vulva.

PUERPERIUM: (*puer* = child; *parere* = to bear) the period of time from delivery to the return of the uterus to its normal size and function.

TOXEMIA OF PREGNANCY: a condition due to metabolic disturbance during pregnancy. *Preeclampsia* and *eclampsia* are the more severe stages.

TRIMESTER: one-third of the period of gestation, i.e., the first three months is the first trimester, the 4th to 6th months the second, and the 7th to 9th the third.

ENDOCRINE SYSTEM

(Specialist practicing in this field is the Endocrinologist)

ANATOMICAL PARTS

ANALYSIS, DEFINITIONS AND NARRATIONS

Example Terms

ADRENAL GLAND: (*ad* = to; *ren* = kidney). This gland is above the kidney and is sometimes called the suprarenal. It secretes at least two hormones: adrenalin and cortin. Adrenalin has a stimulating effect upon the sympathic nerves and gives energy when one is excited by fear or in quick need of energy. This hormone is not considered essential. Cortin is essential to life. It helps regulate the mineral, water and carbohydrate metabolism.

CAROTID GLAND: (*karoun* = to plunge into deep sleep). The name was first given to the arteries of the neck because, when pressed hard, a stupefying effect resulted. These glands are named from the arteries and are placed near the juncture where the carotid arteries branch off.

ENDOCRINE GLAND: (*endon* = within; *krinein* = to separate) a gland which secretes directly into the blood stream, so that its product is widely distributed. Most glands produce substances which are of local importance but are not widely distributed in the body.

GONADS: (*gonos* = semen, seed or generation). The gonads are the seed-producing organs; the ovary and testis.

INSULAR TISSUE: Specific cells in the pancreas which produce the hormone insulin. The hormone insulin is necessary for the metabolism of carbohydrates.

PINEAL GLAND: (*pinea* = pine cone or pineapple). The gland, so called because of its shape, has been called by many other names: parietal body, median eye, third eye, pineal eye, pinus and penis cerebri. It is the organ which prevents too rapid development of the reproductive organs and inhibits sex.

PITUITARY GLAND: (*pituita* = mucus or phlegm secretion). Early anatomists thought that mucus from nose and mouth filtered through the ethmoid from the brain. The word spit is related to this term. Thus the reason for the name pituitary.

Example Terms

The pituitary gland is known to produce at least 5 hormones: the growth hormone, the thyrotropic hormone which stimulates the thyroid, the adrenotropic hormone which stimulates the adrenal gland, the gonadotropic hormone which stimulates the ovary in the female and the testis in the male, and the lactogenic hormone which causes production of milk in female breast tissue. The "master gland."

THYMUS GLAND: (*thymos* = a warty growth, or from *thyme* = a plant, or from *thymos* = soul). Authors disagree on the meaning of this term, and when the authorities disagree, the ignorant may presume. Thyme, a plant, comes from a word meaning to offer, or sacrifice, and was burnt on the sacrificial altars because of its sweet odor. The term may have been applied to the gland because it resembled the wartlike excrescence from the plant, or it may have been taken from the term meaning soul because the gland lies near the heart and our souls were supposed to be closely connected with our hearts. The thymus is a gland lying in the anterior mediastinal cavity. It is concerned with production of lymphocytes in the embryo, with metabolism, growth and development.

THYROID GLAND: (*thyreos* = a large oblong shield; *oid* = like or resemblance to). The term was first used to mean a large stone placed against a door to keep it shut. Later, it was applied to a long shield which covered the length of a soldier. In anatomy, the term was first applied to the cartilage in the neck. The gland got its name from the cartilage. It is the organ which secretes an iodine compound.

CONDITIONS AND DISEASES OF THE ENDOCRINE SYSTEM

ANALYSIS, DEFINITIONS AND NARRATIONS

Example Terms

ACROMEGALY: a disease of the pituitary gland characterized by great enlargement of the hands and feet, the face and lower jaw, and overgrowth of the body hair.

Example Terms

ADENOMATOUS GOITRE: a disease of the thyroid gland with small nodules of thyroid tissue throughout the gland giving it asymmetry.

ADRENAL CORTICAL HYPOFUNCTION: (Addison's disease) a condition in which there is insufficiency of the cortex of the adrenal glands.

ATROPHY OF THYROID GLAND, CONGENITAL: (Cretinism) dwarfism due to deficiency or absence of the thyroid secretion in early childhood. Most cretins are apathetic and sluggish, and there is associated mental deficiency.

DIABETES INSIPIDUS: a disease of the pituitary gland in which large quantities of urine of very low specific gravity and low chloride content are excreted. (Not to be confused with diabetes mellitus.)

DIABETES MELLITUS: (*diabetes* = a syphon; *mellitus* = honey sweet) a disease caused by the insufficiency of the insulin secretion of the pancreas.

DISEASES OF THE PINEAL GLAND: rare, but any condition which destroys the function of the gland results in rapid sexual development and sexual precocity.

DYSTROPHIA ADIPOSOGENITALIS: (Fröhlich's syndrome) (*adeps* = fat) a disease of the pituitary gland characterized by sexual hypoplasia, excessive adiposity, with fat deposits in the breasts, hips and abdominal regions, and other symptoms.

HYPERPARATHYROIDISM: a disease of the parathyroid glands characterized by increase in blood calcium with resultant decalcification of the bones. This may give rise to osteitis fibrosa cystica.

HYPOPITUITARY CACHEXIA: (Simmond's disease) a disease of the pituitary gland characterized by premature senility, loss of axillary and pubic hair, premature gray hair, generalized emaciation and other symptoms.

Example Terms

MYXEDEMA: the result of thyroid deficiency in older children or in adults and similar to the cretinism of children.

PITUITARY BASOPHILISM: a disease of the pituitary gland characterized by obesity of trunk and face, excessive hairiness, cyanosis of face and hands, softening of bones, and other symptoms.

PITUITARY (HYPOPHYSEAL) GIGANTISM: a condition of overgrowth of the skeleton, producing a person of enormous stature with unusually long arms and legs.

TETANY: a condition due to severe lowering of the calcium in the blood, caused when the parathyroid glands are destroyed by disease or surgically removed. (Hyperventilation is another frequent cause.)

THYROIDITIS: inflammation of the thyroid gland.

TOXIC DIFFUSE GOITRE: (*goitre; guttur* = the throat) a condition which shows hypertrophy and hyperplasia of the thyroid gland with decreased iodine in the gland and increased iodine in the blood. Protrusion of the eyeballs is a feature.

TOXIC NODULAR GOITRE: a condition showing the features of exophthalmic goitre with the exception of exophthalmos.

NERVOUS SYSTEM

(The specialist practicing in this field is called a Neurologist and/or Neurosurgeon)

ANATOMICAL PARTS

ANALYSIS, DEFINITIONS AND NARRATIONS

Example Terms

ARACHNOID: (*arachne* = spider; *oid* = resemblance). It means spider-like and is so named because it is a layer covering the brain and spinal cord and is cobweb-like.

Example Terms

AUTONOMIC NERVOUS SYSTEM: (*nomos* = law) the cranial, thoracolumbar, and sacral nerve outflows. The thoracolumbar outflow is the sympathetic nervous system; the two others together are the parasympathetic. Autonomic is here used in the sense of self-controlled or involuntary, i.e., not under conscious control.

BRAIN: (possibly from *brechmos* = forehead; or the Anglo-Saxon term *braegen,* meaning brain). The early Egyptians believed that the brain was the seat of emotion or the abode of the soul. It is the mass of nervous material within the bony skull or cranium (see also *encephalon*).

CAUDA EQUINA: (*cauda* = tail; *equina* = resembling a horse) the roots of the sacral and coccygeal nerves, so named for their resemblance to a horse's tail.

CAVUM SEPTI PELLUCIDI: (*cavus* = hollow; *septum* = partition; *lucere* = to shine) the cavity of the fifth ventricle.

CEREBELLUM: (diminutive of cerebrum) the little brain. It is that part of the brain which coordinates movement.

CEREBRUM: (*cerebrum* = brain) the main portion of the brain.

CISTERNA AMBIENS: (*cisterna* = a reservoir) a pocket of cerebrospinal fluid situated over the optic lobes. Other *cisternae* of the brain are *basalis* and *magna.*

CORPUS CALLOSUM: (*callosus* = hard, thick-skinned) the broad band of white matter uniting the cerebral hemispheres.

CORTEX: (*cortex* = bark or outer layer) the outer layer of an organ, especially the brain.

DURA and PIA MATER: (*dura* = hard; *pia* = soft; *mater* = mother). These are the outer coverings of the brain and spinal cord. The dura was named because it is the tough outer covering; the pia, because it is the soft innermost covering. At one time it was presumed that these membranes, or coverings, were the mother of all body membranes; hence, mater.

Example Terms

EPENDYMA: (*endyma* = a cloak or outer garment) the lining of the cerebral ventricles. Actually the name means the opposite of a lining.

FALX CEREBRI: (*falx* = a sickle) a sickle-shaped fold of the dura mater.

FORAMEN: (*forare* = to bore) an opening, of which there are several in the cranium. The plural of the word is *foramina* or (modern) foramens.

GANGLION: (*ganglion* = a knot or swelling; plural is *ganglia*) a knot of nerve cells. The name originally meant any subcutaneous swelling; now it is applied to any collection of nerve cells that serves as a center for nervous influence.

GASSERIAN GANGLION: the sensory ganglion of the trigeminal nerve (5th cranial nerve).

LEPTOMENINGES: (*leptos* = delicate) the pia mater and arachnoid membranes, which are both thin and delicate. The dura mater is tough and strong.

MEDULLA OBLONGATA: (*medulla* = marrow; *oblongus* = rather long or oblong) the long portion of the brain between the pons and spinal cord.

MENINGES: (*meninx*, plural *meninges* = membrane). This term was first applied to mean all membranes of the body. The constant application of it to the brain and spinal cord caused it finally to be applied only to the coverings of these parts.

NERVE: (*neuron* or *nervus* = tendon or nerve, meaning string). Early anatomists called any band of whitish structure a nerve. It refers now only to nerves, the cordlike structures which convey impulses from one part of the body to another.

OPTIC THALAMUS: (*thalamos* = an inner chamber) a mass of gray matter in the lateral wall of the third ventricle.

Example Terms

PARASAGITTAL: (*sagitta* = arrow; *para* = alongside, parallel with) the cerebral meninges adjacent to the sagittal suture of the skull.

PLEXUS: (from *plectere* = to braid or weave) anything woven together. A tangle of nerves.

PONS: (*pons* = bridge) that part of the brain which connects the other 3 parts: the cerebrum, the cerebellum and medulla oblongata.

SCIATIC NERVE: (*sciaticus*, from Gr. *ischiadikus* = pain in the hip, from *ischios* = the hip) a sensory and motor nerve serving the skin of the leg, muscles of back and thigh, and muscles of leg and foot.

SPLANCHNIC NERVES: (*splanchna* = bowels) sympathetic nerves supplying the viscera.

TENTORIUM: (*tendere* = to stretch; hence a tent) an infolding of the dura mater which covers the cerebellum like a tent.

TRIGEMINAL NERVE: (*trigeminus* = triplet) a motor and sensory nerve in three divisions, ophthalmic, superior and inferior maxillary.

VAGUS: (*vagare* = to wander) a nerve serving the ear, pharynx, larynx, heart, lungs, esophagus, stomach and liver. The name well expresses the extensive distribution of this nerve. Formerly known as the *pneumogastric* nerve.

CONDITIONS AND DISEASES OF THE NERVOUS SYSTEM

ANALYSIS, DEFINITIONS AND NARRATIONS

Example Terms

ACUTE ANTERIOR POLIOMYELITIS: (infantile paralysis) believed to be a virus disease. The spinal cord is more severely involved than the brain. The motor cells are the chief victims, hence the danger of paralysis.

Example Terms

CEREBRAL HEMORRHAGE: a condition caused by the rupture of a vessel in the brain, often expressed as "cerebral accident."

CONCUSSION OF THE BRAIN: the shaking and vibration of the brain at the time of a sudden blow on the head, with or without fracture of the skull, resulting in dizziness, nausea, weak pulse, slow respiration and often a loss of consciousness.

CONTUSION OF THE BRAIN: a bruising of the brain substance as a result of trauma. It is usually accompanied by fracture and hemorrhage into the brain.

ENCEPHALITIS: any inflammation of the brain. Some of the types of encephalitis are suppurative (brain abscess), virus (from the virus of poliomyelitis, rabies, etc.), postinfectious (following mumps, measles and smallpox), and traumatic.

ENCEPHALOCELE: a protrusion containing brain tissue.

ENCEPHALOMALACIA: a softening of the brain due to a thrombus or embolus in an artery supplying the brain tissue.

ENCEPHALOPATHY: changes in the brain cells without inflammation.

HERPES ZOSTER (SHINGLES): (*herpo* = I creep; *zoster* = a girdle) disease due to an inflammation of the dorsal root nerve ganglia, but the external manifestations are confined to the skin, an ulcerative rash being distributed over the areas supplied by the involved nerves. ("Shingles" is said to be derived from *cingulum* = a belt or girdle.)

HYDROCEPHALUS: a condition (frequently congenital) characterized by the presence of an excessive amount of spinal fluid within the cranial cavity.

LACERATION OF THE BRAIN: tearing of the brain substance, e.g., by gunshot or stab injury, or skull fracture with bone displacement.

LEPTOMENINGITIS: inflammation of the pia mater and arachnoid, which can be caused by numerous organisms.

Example Terms

MICROCEPHALY: an abnormally small cerebrum in a small skull.

NEURITIS: any sensory or motor disturbance along the distribution of a nerve. It is usually inflammatory, but not invariably so.

PACHYMENINGITIS: inflammation of the dura mater.

SPINAL CORD INJURIES: if severe, they cause paralysis of the extremities supplied by the nerves distal to the site of injury.

TABES DORSALIS: (*tabes* = wasting) a degeneration of fibers in the posterior columns of the spinal cord.

SPECIAL SENSES

ACOUSTIC SENSE: (*akoustikos* = pertains to sound or hearing) the sense of hearing.

GUSTATORY SENSE: (*gustare* = to taste) the sense of taste.

OLFACTORY SENSE: (*olere* = to smell; *facere* = to make) the sense of smell.

VISION: the sense of sight.

SENSE OF VISION

(The specialist practicing in this field is called an Ophthalmologist)

ANATOMICAL PARTS

ANALYSIS, DEFINITIONS AND NARRATIONS

Example Terms

AQUEOUS: (*aqua* = water) the fluid part of the eye filling the chambers in front of the lens; sometimes called the aqueous humor.

CANTHI: (*kanthos* = corner of the eye) the slits or angles of the eye where the lids come together.

Example Terms

CARUNCLE: (*caro* = flesh; plus the diminutive *unculus,* hence a small bit of flesh) any small fleshy body. It is the small red eminence in the inner corner, the *caruncle lacrimalis.*

CHOROID: In the eye, it refers to the posterior portion of the middle coat of the eyeball.

CONJUNCTIVA: (*con* = with; *jungere* = to join) the membrane which connects the eyeball with the lids; the lining of the eyelids.

CORNEA: (*corneus* = horny), prefix is *kerato* (from *keras* = horn). The front part of the external layer of the eyeball.

EYEBALL: globe or ball of eye; prefix is *ophthalmo.*

IRIS: (*iris* = rainbow) the pigmented part which encloses the pupil of the eye. The messenger from the gods to man, who came down the rainbow to deliver his message, was called Iris. It is so called because of its varied hues.

LACRIMAL GLANDS and DUCTS: (*lacrima* = a tear) the tear-producing glands and reservoir which holds them; alternatively called (Greek) dacryocyst.

LENS: (*lens* = lentil, an edible plant) so called because it is shaped like the lentil seed. The lens is a transparent substance in the eye shaped to focus light rays.

LIMBUS (of the cornea) : (*limbus* = a border) the edge of the cornea where it meets the sclerotic coat.

MEIBOMIAN GLANDS: (Heinrich Meibom, 1638-1700, a German anatomist) small glands on the inner surface of the eyelids which secrete an oily liquid that keeps the lids from sticking together.

ORBIT: (*orbis* = a ring or circle) the bony socket which contains the eye.

Example Terms

RETINA: (*rete* = a net) the delicate terminal expansion of the optic nerve, upon which light is focussed by the lens. There is no good explanation of the origin of this name. A word meaning a fisherman's net has gradually come to be applied to the sensitive part of the eye which receives the images. But like a net, it gathers in many things.

SCLERA: (*skleros* = hard) the hard outer layer of the eye.

STROMA (of the cornea) : (*stroma* = a mattress) the basic or framework tissue of the cornea.

TARSUS: (*tarsos* = a crate or wicker basket; a framework) the framework which gives shape to the eyelid.

UVEAL TRACT: (*uva* = a grape) the pigmented middle layer of the eye, the iris, ciliary body and choroid.

VITREOUS: (noun, *vitrum* = glass; adjective *vitreus* = glassy). The gelatinous matter which fills the posterior chamber of the eye behind the lens; sometimes referred to as vitreous humor.

CONDITIONS AND DISEASES OF SENSE OF VISION

ANALYSIS, DEFINITIONS AND NARRATIONS

Example Terms

ACHROMATOPSIA: color blindness.

CATARACT: (*cata* = down; *arassein* = to dash; hence a waterfall, also a portcullis) an opacity of the lens or its capsule.

CHALAZION: (*chalaza* = a hailstone) inflammation of a Meibomian gland which forms a tumorlike rise of the lid.

CONJUNCTIVITIS: inflammation of the conjunctiva.

ECTROPION : eversion of the eyelid margin.

ENTROPION: inversion of the eyelid margin.

HYPERMETROPIA : farsightedness.

Example Terms

IRIDOCYCLITIS: inflammation of the iris and ciliary body.

MYOPIA: nearsightedness.

NYSTAGMUS: a rhythmic oscillation of the eyeballs.

RETINAL DETACHMENT: detachment of a portion of the retina, usually due to trauma.

STRABISMUS: (*strabismos* = squinting) "cross-eye."

SENSE OF HEARING

(The specialist practicing in this field is called an Otologist or Otorhinolaryngologist because of the Ear, Nose and Throat combination)

ANATOMICAL PARTS

ANALYSIS, DEFINITIONS AND NARRATIONS

Example Terms

COCHLEA: (*cochlea* = a snail) a spiral-shaped bony hollow of the internal ear.

EAR: prefix is *oto* or *audio* or *auri* (*auris* = ear) the organ of hearing.

EUSTACHIAN TUBE: (Bartolommeo Eustachio, 1520-1574, Italian anatomist) the auditory tube connecting the pharynx with the tympanic cavity.

LABYRINTH: the small maze of canals of the inner ear, containing endolymph, the movement of which causes variations of pressure which are "measured" by the brain and has a function of maintaining balance.

MASTOID AIR CELLS: (*mastos* = breast; *oid* = like) a cavity shaped like a breast. An outgrowth or process of cavities of the temporal bone.

Example Terms

OSSEOUS MEATUS: (*osteon* or *os* = bone; meatus from *meare* = to go or pass) a bony channel or passageway. Here it refers to the external canal of the hearing organ.

PETROUS PORTION: (*petra* = a rock) the "stony" or solid part of the temporal bone.

SACCULE: (*sac* = a bag) the smaller of two saclike structures of the inner ear.

SEMICIRCULAR CANAL: (*semi* = half) one of the small canals of the labyrinth.

TYMPANIC MEMBRANE: (*tympanum* = drum or tambourine) membrane stretched across the opening of the middle ear; the ear drum.

UTRICLE: (diminutive of uterus) the larger of two saclike structures of the inner ear.

VESTIBULAR EQUILIBRATORY SENSE: (*vestibulum* = a forecourt or antechamber; *equi* = equal; *libra* = balance or level) the sense which maintains balance.

CONDITIONS AND DISEASES OF SENSE OF HEARING

ANALYSIS, DEFINITIONS AND NARRATIONS

Example Terms

MASTOIDITIS: inflammation of the mastoid cells. It frequently follows otitis media.

MÉNIÈRE'S DISEASE: a combination of symptoms, viz., vertigo, nausea, tinnitus and progressive deafness, usually due to hemorrhage, edema or vasospasm in the semicircular canals.

OTALGIA: earache.

OTITIS (MEDIA, INTERNA, EXTERNA): inflammation of the ear (middle, inner, external).

Example Terms

TINNITUS: (*tinnitus* = a tinkling sound) "ringing in the ears," a sensation caused by irritation of the auditory nerve.

VERTIGO: (*vertere* = to turn) "dizziness," a disorder of equilibrium resulting from disease of the middle ear, also from cardiac, gastric, central nervous system and ocular disorders. True vertigo is when the surroundings spin. Dizziness is more a feeling of faintness.

Chapter VIII

MEDICAL RECORDS AND
WORDS COMMONLY FOUND IN THEM

Part I

A. Analysis of Words

B. Sample Exercises

Part II

The Medical Record

(Courtesy of Duke University School of Medicine. From "Medical Records: Composition, Procedures and Policies," written for classroom instruction by JeHarned.)

ANALYSIS OF WORDS

A MEDICAL record is defined as a clear, concise and accurate history of the patient's life and illness, written from the medical point of view. Unless medical jargon in shortened terminology were employed to express numerous disease conditions, the medical record in its completed form would cover many more pages. A patient may say, in nonmedical language, that he has a constant craving for water which he cannot satisfy; the physician writes the one word *polydipsia* to express the same condition. Or, the patient may state that his hair is falling out in patches and he has bald spots all over his head; the physician expresses the same condition in the term *alopecia areata*. If a mother states that she has been pregnant five times, has lost one pregnancy by miscarriage and has four living children, the physician writes in the record *para: 5-1-4*. The parts of the medical record called the History and Physical Examination abound in these terms.

This chapter contains an alphabetical list of many medical terms commonly found in medical records as well as an outline of data which are necessary in the composition of a medical record. Analysis of the words, part by part, is given here as well as the definition, but further help is presented by showing an example of use of terms as the medically trained person may employ them.

Since the beginner in medical terminology has, up to this point, learned stems and affixes as well as the formula of defining a word by analysis of its meaningful parts, instruction beginning with this chapter might be called an advanced course. The student may now be permitted to concentrate on exercises showing proper use of terms. Sample exercises are included to help the instructor and student.

Word	Analysis	Meaning	Example of Use
ABASIA	a = neg.; basis = step	Not able to walk.	Paralysis of the leg is a cause of abasia.
ABDUCT	ab = from; ducere = to draw	To draw away from.	Abduct the leg to determine ability of outward motion.
ABERRANT	ab = from; errare = to stray	Straying or wandering from the normal course.	An aberrant blood vessel.
ABRASION	ab = from; radere = to scrape	Rubbed or scraped off (the word razor comes from radere).	Abrasions of skin may result from too vigorous use of a razor.
ACARIASIS	acarus = mite; iasis = condition	State or condition of being infested with mites.	Acariasis of scalp.
ACETONE	acetum = vinegar	A liquid sometimes found in considerable quantity in the urine of diabetic persons.	Acetone bodies.
ACHALASIA	a = neg.; chalasis = relaxation	Failure to relax.	Achalasia of sphincter of esophagus.

Word	Analysis	Meaning	Example of Use
ACHOLURIA	a = without; chole = bile; ouron = urine	Absence of bile pigment in urine.	Acholuria is symptomatic of a type of jaundice.
ACUTE	acutus = sharp	It expresses a severe and relatively short course of illness.	Acute abdominal pain.
ADDUCT	ad = toward; ducere = to draw	To draw toward.	Adduct the leg to determine ability of motion toward the body.
ADENTIA	a = without; dens = tooth	Without teeth.	Examination of mouth shows complete adentia.
ADIPOSE	adeps = fat	Fatty.	Adipose tissue.
ADNEXA	ad = to; nectere = to bind or join	Structures attached to each other or accessory parts adjoining. (Annexa is often used instead of adnexa.)	The adnexa uteri are the ovaries and oviducts.
AERO-PHAGIA	aer = air; phagein = to eat	Swallowing air.	Aerophagia is frequently present in hysteria.
AGENESIS	a = without; genesis = generation	Not produced or absent at birth.	Agenesis of kidney or any organ.

Word	Analysis	Meaning	Example of Use
AGERASIA	*a* = neg.; *geras* = old age	Young appearance in old age.	Agerasia of a patient 70 years of age.
AKINESIA (ak-in-e′se-ah)	*a* = neg.; *kinesis* = movement	Absence or weakness of motor function.	Temporary paralysis produced by injection of procaine is a type of akinesia.
ALBU- MINURIA	*albumin* = protein; *ouron* = urine	Protein in urine.	Urinalysis showed albuminuria.
ALEXIA	*a* = neg.; *lexis* = speaking	Word blindness.	A patient having motor alexia may understand what he sees but is unable to read it aloud.
ALOPECIA (al-o-pe′she-ah)	*alopex* = fox	This is a very old term which may have come into use because of several reasons. It was noticed that where the fox urinated, the earth would be barren; or, a head which became partially bald looked like a mangy fox. Baldness.	Alopecia areata or baldness in patches.

Word	Analysis	Meaning	Example of Use
AMBLYOPIA	amblys = dull; opia = sight	Dimness of vision.	On examination of the eyes, the patient showed no sign of amblyopia.
AMBULANT	ambulare = to walk about	Able to walk; not confined to bed.	A patient may be ambulant.
AMPHIBOLIA	amphibolos = doubtful	In medical use it refers to uncertainty or vacillating period of outcome of a disease; doubtful prognosis.	Changing fever during a disease may be the period of amphibolia.
ANALGESIA	an = neg.; algos = pain; ia = condition of	Painless or absence of feeling pain.	By pin prick, the patient shows complete analgesia on the left arm.
ANESTHESIA	an = neg.; esthesia = condition of feeling	No feeling or loss of feeling.	A patient may complain of anesthesia of a part; or, general anesthesia was produced by administration of ether and oxygen.
ANEURYSM	ana =across or through; eurys = broad	Broad across; a widening or dilatation.	Aneurysm of an artery.

Word	Analysis	Meaning	Example of Use
ANGINA	*angere* = to strangle or throttle	In the beginning of the use of this term it was applied to mean a sore throat or anything which caused an obstruction of the larynx. It has therefore come to mean a choking sensation or pain which causes suffocation.	An attack of angina may mean a serious heart disease.
ANGIOMA	*angeion* = vessel; *oma* = tumor	Tumor whose cells seem to form blood vessels.	Angioma (synonymous with hemangioma) of conjunctiva.
ANISOCORIA	*aniso* = unequal; *corê* = pupil	Unequal pupils.	Anisocoria is often an hereditary trait.
ANISOPIA	*aniso* = unequal; *opia* = vision	Unequal vision in the two eyes.	Special eyeglasses are prescribed for anisopia.
ANKYLOSIS	*ankylos* = bent or crooked; *osis* = condition of	Although this word means crooked, it has come to be used in the sense that it is a fixed crookedness, or stiffness with crookedness.	The elbow shows a 30-degree ankylosis.
ANOMALY	*an* = not or neg.; *homalos* = even	An irregularity or something out of the ordinary or not normal.	A child with six fingers has an anomaly.

Word	Analysis	Meaning	Example of Use
ANOREXIA	*an* = without; *orexis* = appetite	Loss of appetite.	The patient is weak due to anorexia.
ANOXIA	*an* = without; *oxygène* = oxygen; *ia* = condition	Oxygen deficiency.	Anoxia may occur at high altitudes.
ANTHRACOSIS	*anthrax* = coal; *osis* = condition	An accumulation of coal dust in the lungs.	Melanoptysis may be a symptom of anthracosis.
ANURIA	*an* = neg.; *ouron* = urine	Suppression of urine in kidney.	Uremia is a result of anuria.
AORTOLITH	*aorta* = large artery which suspends the heart; *lithos* = stone or calculus	Calculus formation on walls of aorta.	An aortolith may show up on x-ray examination.
APEX	*apex* = tip end or top; pl. = *apices*	The upper or pointed end.	The apex of the lung was dull to percussion.
APHASIA	*a* = without; *phasis* = utterance	Unable to speak.	Because of a tumor of the larynx, the patient has constant aphasia.

Word	Analysis	Meaning	Example of Use
APHONIA	a = without; phoné = voice	Loss of voice.	Aphonia is often due to paralysis of the vocal cords.
APLASIA	a = without; plasis = molding or forming	Not formed.	Aplasia of the bone marrow may cause a person to appear pale.
APNEA	a = not; pneo = I breathe	Breathlessness.	Apnea may follow overexertion.
APRAXIA	a = neg.; praxis = doing	Purposeless movement; loss of ability to perform purposefully; mind blindness.	Apraxia as a sequela of brain pathology.
ASCITES	askos = a sac or bladder	Since a bag or sac is filled with fluid, this word has come to mean fluid in the peritoneal sac or abdominal cavity.	Paracentesis of abdomen may be done to relieve ascites.
ASEPSIS	a = not; sepsis = decay or infection	A condition of being free of infection.	To practice asepsis is to keep free of disease and infection.
ASTHENIA	a = without; sthenos = strength	Weakness.	Because of anorexia, a patient may suffer loss of weight and generalized asthenia.

Word	Analysis	Meaning	Example of Use
ATHEROMA	*athêrê* = gruel or porridge; *oma* = tumor	This word may be used to mean two things: it may mean a tumorous mass of the consistency of porridge, such as a sebaceous cyst, or it may mean a thickened condition or change in the walls of the arteries.	On the skin were found many small atheromata. Arteriosclerosis with marked changes in the vessel walls is often called an atheromatous condition.
ATHETOSIS	*a* = not; *thetos* = fixed or stationary	A slow involuntary movement of hands and feet, especially in children.	A patient suffering from certain brain diseases may develop athetosis.
ATONY	*a* = without; *tonos* = tone or strength	Want of normal tone or vital energy.	Atony of uterus causes a difficult labor. Atony of muscles.
ATRESIA	*a* = not; *tresis* = boring	Not open; closure of a normal opening.	An imperforate anus may be described as complete or partial atresia.
ATROPHY	*a* = without; *trophe* = nourishment	Not fed, or undersized.	Atrophy of any organ may mean that it has never grown to a normal size or has wasted away.

Word	Analysis	Meaning	Example of Use
AUSCULTA-TION	*auscultare* = to listen intently or hear	One of the oldest methods of examination of a patient was to place the ear against the chest to listen to breathing and the heart beat. This is direct auscultation. With the invention of the stethoscope, this type of examination is now done by indirect auscultation.	By auscultation, the breathing was heard to be of a rasping nature and the heart beat rapid.
AUTOGE-NOUS	*auto* = self ; *genos* = origin	Originating in or generated by one's self.	Vaccines are often made from the germs of a patient himself. Therefore, an autogenous vaccine is one made for a patient from his own infection.
AUTOPSY	*auto* = self ; *opsis* = seeing	The original meaning of this term was self-seeing, or seeing for one's self. In other words, it meant examination by the physician himself. At the present time it is restricted to mean dissection of a dead body.	When we speak of a post-mortem examination, we mean an autopsy was done.

Word	Analysis	Meaning	Example of Use
BABINSKI	*Joseph Babinski* = a French neurologist	Babinski reflex is an abnormal reaction of the toes when the sole of the foot is stroked. The toes extend out, especially the great toe.	To express this condition, the physician states that the Babinski is present. The presence of the Babinski indicates a disease of the spinal cord. If the physician states that the Babinski is absent, the toes have reacted normally to stroking and have curled under.
BACILLUS	diminutive of *baculum* = a rod; pl. = *bacilli*	A rod-shaped germ.	A culture may show *Bacillus coli.*
BACTERIUM	diminutive of *baktron* = a cane or staff; pl. = *bacteria*	A minute staff-shaped animal or plant seen only under a microscope, which may cause disease. Bacteria are preferably called microorganisms.	Bacteria are isolated in a culture of pus.

Word	Analysis	Meaning	Example of Use
BALLOTTE-MENT	ballotter = to toss about; ment = a suffix to form a noun implying action	To toss about like a bouncing ball.	Ballottement is a sharp upward pushing against the uterine wall with the finger, for diagnosing pregnancy by feeling the return impact of the displaced fetus. A similar procedure of ballottement may be performed to diagnose a floating kidney.
BIFURCA-TION	bi = two; furca = fork	A main stem branching off into two forks or branches.	The abdominal aorta is bifurcated. A clot of blood could be lodged at this bifurcation.
BLOOD PRESSURE	premere = to press	The pressure of blood on the walls of the arteries.	Blood pressure may be expressed as 140/80.
BORBORYG-MUS (bor-bo-rig'mus)	borborygmus = rumbling noise	A rumbling of the bowels.	Borborygmi are frequently heard in intestinal obstruction.
BRADY-CARDIA	brady = slow; cardia = heart	A slow heart beat.	Examination by auscultation may show a bradycardia.

Word	Analysis	Meaning	Example of Use
BRADYPNEA	*brady* = slow; *pneo* = I breathe	Slow breathing.	Bradypnea is a symptom of many diseases.
BREECH	*brec* = an Anglo-Saxon word used for clothing which covered the lower trunk and thighs; a pair of britches	The buttocks.	Breech presentation is when the buttocks appear first in the birth of a child.
BRUIT	*bruit* = noise	A word used to denote abnormal sounds, murmurs, and various other noises in the chest.	On auscultation, bruits can be heard throughout the chest.
CACHEXIA (kak-eks'e-ah)	*kakos* = ill or bad; *hexis* = condition of body	General debility or ill health with malnutrition.	On examination, a patient may be found to be in a state of cachexia if he has a wasting disease like cancer.
CANCER	*cancer* = a crab	A malignant growth or tumor.	Cancer is the layman's word for carcinoma.
CARIES	*caries* = dry rot	Used to indicate the decay of bonelike structures when they become softened, discolored, porous and fetid.	Caries of the teeth.

Word	Analysis	Meaning	Example of Use
CARPHO-LOGIA	*karphos* = chaff or nesting material; *logia* = collection	A word used to indicate involuntary picking at bed clothes when a patient is feverish and delirious.	Carphologia is sometimes noted during the stuporous condition of the patient.
CATHARSIS	*katharsis* = cleansing; purification	A purgation of the bowels.	Catharsis is given in constipation.
CATHETER	*katheter* = something sent down	A tube sent down a passage for the purpose of feeding or draining.	To force-feed a patient a catheter is used through the nose, entering into the esophagus. To relieve the contents of the urinary bladder a catheter is inserted through the urethra into the bladder.
CAU-SALGIA	*kausis* = burning; *algos* = pain	A burning pain.	Causalgia of face following "stroke."
CEPHA-LALGIA	*cephale* = head; *algos* = pain	A headache.	Cephalalgia is a forerunner of many diseases.
CERUMEN	*cera* = wax	Earwax.	Impacted cerumen.
CHIROPO-DALGIA (ki-ro-po-dal′-je-ah)	*chiro* = hand; *pous* = foot; *algos* = pain	Pain in hands and feet.	Chiropodalgia as a result of nerve pathology.

Word	Analysis	Meaning	Example of Use
CHOREA	*choreia* = a dance	Uncontrolled jerking movements and twitchings. In the 15th century a peculiar type of dance came into vogue which developed into maniacal proportions. People danced for hours until they worked themselves into throes of mental agitation and fell to the ground foaming at the mouth. Some of these people twitched and jerked in a faint. When the dance reached epidemic characteristics, the magistrate ordered such persons to the chapel of St. Vitus. St. Vitus prayed that persons commemorating the date of his death would not be afflicted. Convulsive twitchings in real diseases came then to be known as St. Vitus' dance and later as chorea.	Chorea usually occurs in early life.

Word	Analysis	Meaning	Example of Use
CHRONIC	*chronos* = time	Anything of long duration; the opposite of acute.	An ache which lasts over a period of time signifies a chronic disease.
CICATRIX (sik-a'triks)	*cicare* = to form a skin over	A scar.	A wound heals and a cicatrix forms.
CLAUDICA-TION	*claudicare* = to limp	Lameness or walking with a limp. In medicine it signifies pain caused by spasm of an artery.	Intermittent claudication is marked in the left leg.
CLIMAC-TERIC	*klimax* = a stair-case or ladder; *klimakter* = a step of the stairway or rung of the ladder	The ancients considered that life changed every seven years. It was called a climacteric because it was another rung up on the ladder of life. The greatest change or grand climacteric was supposed to come about the 63rd year of life. The word now signifies menopause or "change of life" in women.	The climacteric is a normal phenomenon but is sometimes associated with irritability, nervousness and headache.

Word	Analysis	Meaning	Example of Use
CLINICIAN	*kliné* = bed	One who practices at the bed-side. A physician who is distinguished from those who do laboratory work.	A clinician makes the bedside diagnosis.
CLONUS	*klonos* = a turmoil	A spasm or irregular muscular contraction.	On examination of reflexes of a patient, ankle clonus may be noted. It is induced by suddenly pushing up the foot while the leg is extended. Result of the sudden push is several convulsive movements of the ankle. If ankle clonus is present, it indicates disease of certain parts of the brain or spinal cord.
COITION	*coitus* = going together	Sexual intercourse.	Painful coition.
COLIC	*kolikos* = relating to colon	Severe griping pain.	Kidney colic or intestinal colic.

Word	Analysis	Meaning	Example of Use
COMA	*koma* = deep sleep	Unconsciousness.	A patient is in coma or a comatose condition if he cannot be aroused by external stimuli.
CONGENITAL	*con* = with; *genitus* = born	A thing present at birth, not necessarily hereditary.	Harelip is a congenital cleft of the lip.
CORONER	*corona* = crown	The term now refers to a person who investigates cases of sudden death.	A death certificate may be issued or revoked by a coroner's decision.
CREPITUS	*crepitare* = to crackle	Crackling noise.	Crepitus is noticed in grating of fractured bones, the crackling of joints, the noise produced by pressure on tissues containing excessive air or gas; or, crepitant rales of the chest may be heard on auscultation.
CUL-DE-SAC	*cul* = bottom; *de* = of; *sac* = bag	Bottom of a bag or a blind passage.	On examination of the rectum a hard mass was found in the cul-de-sac.
CULTURE	*cultura* = a growth	In medicine this applies to an artificial growth of bacteria.	A culture is made from pus from an abscess to learn the type of bacteria causing the infection.

Word	Analysis	Meaning	Example of Use
CYANOSIS	kyanos = blue; osis = a condition of	A condition of blueness of the skin produced by lack of oxygen. It means usually the patient is not breathing deeply.	The fingers, nose and tips of the ears show cyanosis in pneumonia.
DECUBITUS	decumbere = to lie down	The recumbent position; bed-sore caused from lying abed in prolonged illness.	A decubitus ulcer.
DEFECATION	de = away from; faex = dregs	Removal of dregs or bowel movement.	On defecation, blood may be noticed in the stool.
DEGLUTI-TION	glutire = to swallow	Swallowing.	Deglutition may be forced by gentle pressure on the throat.
DEHYDRA-TION	de = away; hydor = water	A condition resulting from loss of water from tissues.	Dehydration may result from high fevers.
DESQUAMA-TION	de = from; squama = a scale	A shedding of outer layers, as a peeling skin.	Any rash may be in the process of desquamation.
DIAGNOSIS	dia = through; gnosis = knowledge; pl. = diagnoses	A conclusion reached. In medicine, it is naming the disease.	After thorough examination, the doctor made a diagnosis of tuberculosis.
DIAPHORE-SIS	dia = through; phorea = I carry	Profuse perspiration.	Diaphoresis, as a symptom in tuberculosis.

Word	Analysis	Meaning	Example of Use
DIFFUSE	*dis* = apart; *fundere* = to pour or scatter	Widely scattered; not localized.	Diffuse cracklings were heard throughout the lungs.
DIPLEGIA	*di* = two; *plege* = stroke	A paralysis affecting both sides alike.	Cerebral hemorrhage may result in diplegia.
DORSAL	*dorsum* = the back; pl.= *dorsa*	Relates to position, the back side.	The dorsal part of the hand is opposite the palm.
DYSKINESIA	*dys* = difficult; *kinesis* = movement	Impairment of power of voluntary movement.	Dyskinesia following cerebral vascular accident.
DYSLALIA	*dys* = difficult; *lalia* = talking	Speech defect.	Lisping is a form of dyslalia.
DYSLEXIA	*dys* = difficult; *lexis* = diction; *ia* = condition	Inability to read under-standingly.	Children with a dyslexia trait often must have special tutoring in reading.
DYS-PAREUNIA	*dys* = difficult; *pareunos* = lying beside	Painful intercourse.	Dyspareunia is a word frequent-ly found in histories of gyne-cological patients.

Word	Analysis	Meaning	Example of Use
DYSPHAGIA	dys = difficult or painful; phagein = to eat	Painful swallowing.	Following removal of tonsils, a patient may suffer dysphagia.
DYSPHEMIA	dys = difficult; pheme = speech	Stammering.	Psychologists sometimes suggest that dysphemia may be corrected by parents who ignore its presence.
DYSPHONIA	dys = difficult or painful; phonia = act of speaking	Difficulty of speech.	A tongue-tied person has dysphonia.
DYSPLASIA	dys = ill; plasis = form	Ill-formed or undeveloped.	Smallness of the internal organs is one form of dysplasia.
DYSPNEA	dys = difficult or painful; pnea = breathing	Difficult or painful breathing.	One cause of dyspnea may be asthma.
DYSTOCIA	dys = difficult or painful; tokos = birth or labor	Difficult birth of a child.	Dystocia in prolonged labor.

Word	Analysis	Meaning	Example of Use
ECLAMPSIA	ec = out from; lampo = I shine or flash	To flash out or break forth suddenly. At one time this word indicated a sudden fever. It has come to mean presence of poisons in the system during pregnancy: toxemia of pregnancy. This name was probably so called because of its sudden onset with convulsions.	Precautions against eclampsia may be taken by rest and quiet.
ECTOPIC	ec = out; topos = place	A thing which is out of place.	A pregnancy which grows outside the uterus is ectopic.
ECTROPION	ec = out; trope = a turning	An outward turning.	Ectropion of the eyelid.
EDEMA	oidema = a swelling	This term is used to indicate a collection of fluid in the tissues. Dropsy is the lay term.	Pitting of the ankles is an indication of edema.
EDENTU-LOUS	e = without; dens = tooth	Without teeth.	An edentulous mouth.
EMACIATION	emaciare = to become lean	Wasting away.	Emaciation may be a result of cancer.

Word	Analysis	Meaning	Example of Use
EMBOLUS	embolos = a plug; pl. = emboli	A clot of blood, clump of fat, or air bubble which circulates and lodges in a blood vessel, causing obstruction.	Pulmonary embolus.
EMOLLIENT	e = out; mollis = soft	A softening or soothing agent.	Starch may be used as an external emollient, while forms of gelatin are used internally as emollients.
ENDEMIC	en = in; demos = the people	Used to denote disease prevalent in people in a localized region.	Hyperthyroidism is endemic in certain northern states.
ENOPHTHAL-MOS	en = in; ophthalmos = eye	A condition in which the eye sinks back into the socket further than normal.	Enophthalmos may follow an infection of the orbital tissues.
ENTROPION	en = in; trope = a turning	A turning inward.	If the eyelids roll inward, it is called an entropion.
ENURESIS	en = in; ourein = to urinate	Bed-wetting.	Scolding a child at bedtime often brings on enuresis.
EPIDEMIC	epi = upon; demos = the people	A plague on the people; a disease attacking many people in a wide area.	An epidemic of influenza.

Word	Analysis	Meaning	Example of Use
ERUCTATION	*eructare* = to belch	Belching.	Gastric neurosis may be accompanied by eructation.
ETHNICS	*ethnic* = pertains to races of men	Study of races.	Ethnics (or ethnology) may be the hereditary factor in many diseases.
ETIOLOGY	*aitia* = cause; *logos* = study of	The study of causation of disease; the conclusions reached by such study.	The codes in Standard Nomenclature of Disease show placement and etiology of disease.
EUPNEA	*eu* = easy or well; *pnea* = breathing	Easy or normal breathing.	Eupnea is not consistent in asthma.
EXOPHTHALMOS	*ex* = out; *ophthalmos* = eye	Bulging out of eye or protrusion.	Unilateral exophthalmos may indicate a tumor.
EXPECTORATION	*ex* = out; *pectus* = chest	Coughing and spitting out material from air passages.	Expectoration of bloody foam.
EXUDATE	*ex* = out; *sudare* = to sweat	Drainage or fluid which has oozed out.	Considerable amount of exudate may be the result of infection.
FAUCES	*fauces* = the throat passage	Upper part of the throat.	Fauces may be injected.
FEBRILE	*febris* = fever	Feverish.	Being afebrile indicates no fever.

Word	Analysis	Meaning	Example of Use
FECES	*faex* = dregs	Excrement.	The feces of a newborn are called *meconium*.
FETUS	*fetus* = unborn offspring	Child in uterus after the third month.	The heartbeat of the fetus is very rapid.
FISSURE	*fissura* = a cleft or groove; a deep fold	A normal or abnormal groove or cleft in the anatomical makeup.	An infected anal fissure is an abnormal condition, while fissures of the brain are normal folds or grooves.
FISTULA	*fistula* = tube; pl. = *fistulae*	An abnormal passageway between two hollow parts or extending to an external surface of the body.	Fistulae may be caused by infections or created by injury.
FLACCID	*flaccidus* = weak; lax; soft	Laxity of muscle tone, usually soft; flabby.	A flaccid paralysis of a muscle may be the result of poliomyelitis.
FLATUS FLATULENCE	*flatus* = puff of wind	Distention of stomach caused by gas.	Flatulence is often a result of wrong eating.
FOCI OF INFECTION	*focus* = fireplace	Seat of the infection or central point of fire.	Diseased tonsils may be the focus (seat) of infection in iritis.

Word	Analysis	Meaning	Example of Use
FORNIX	*fornix* = arch; pl. = *fornices*	A vaultlike space.	Anterior fornix is the recess between the cervix uteri and anterior wall of vagina.
FOSSA	*fossa* = a ditch; pl. = *fossae*	Depressed areas on body.	The cubital fossa is the depressed area at the elbow.
FOUR-CHETTE	*fourchette* = fork	A fold of mucous membrane at the posterior joining of the labia majora.	Laceration of fourchette often occurs during labor.
FRACTURE	*fractura* = break or rupture	Used to denote a broken bone.	Types of fractures are: Simple fracture = not penetrating the skin. Compound fracture = comes through skin to outside. Incomplete fracture = splintered. Greenstick fracture = splintered. Complete fracture = completely broken across. Comminuted fracture = 3 or more places. Sprain fracture = ligament and bone torn off.

Word	Analysis	Meaning	Example of Use
FREMITUS	*fremitus* = a vibration, roar or murmuring noise	Noises or vibrations which are perceptible when hand is laid on body.	Vocal fremitus in chest is elicited by placing hand on chest when the patient speaks.
FUNDUS	*fundus* = base or bottom part	The fundus is that part of a hollow organ which is furthest away from its external opening.	Fundus of the uterus is that part furthest from the cervix; of the stomach, nearest to the mouth.
GENU	*genu* = knee; pl. = *genua*	Usually refers to knee, but can mean any structure bent like a knee.	Genu varum is bowlegs.
GEOPHAGIA	*ge* = earth; *phagein* = to eat	The habit of eating earth or clay.	A person who forms a habit of eating clay would be a geophagist.
GESTATION	*gestare* = to carry or bear	Pregnancy.	An ectopic gestation is a pregnancy which occurs outside the uterus.
GLABROUS	*glaber* = smooth	Smooth and bare.	Lesion of glabrous skin (means on a part away from places where hair normally grows in thickness).

Word	Analysis	Meaning	Example of Use
HALLUCINA-TION	*hallucinari* = to wander in mind	A word used to indicate that a patient is sensing things which are not real.	Hallucinations of hearing or seeing.
HEMATO-CHEZIA (hem″at-o-ke′ze-ah)	*haima* = blood; *chezein* = to go to stool	Blood in the stool.	Hematochezia is indication for a thorough examination of the intestinal tract.
HEMATURIA	*haima* = blood; *ouron* = urine	Blood in the urine.	A urinalysis may show hematuria.
HEMI-ANOPSIA	*hemi* = half; *an* = not; *opsia* = vision	Half-blind; having sight in only one-half of the field of vision.	Examination of visual fields may show hemianopsia.
HEMOP-TYSIS (hem-op′tis-is)	*haima* = blood; *ptysis* = spitting	Expectoration of blood.	Hemoptysis may be the first symptom of tuberculosis.
HIRSUTISM	*hirsutus* = shaggy; hairy	Abnormally hairy.	A growth of beard on a woman is a feature of hirsutism.
HORMONE	*hormaein* = to excite or arouse	A substance which is produced by one organ and transported to another to cause a specific effect.	Hormone substances found in the pituitary gland which act on other endocrine glands.

Word	Analysis	Meaning	Example of Use
HYDRO-CEPHALUS (hi-dro-sef'-ah-lus)	hydor = water; cephale = head	Abnormal increase in cerebral fluid.	Hydrocephalus may be acquired or a congenital factor.
HYGROMA	hygro = moist; oma = tumor	Usually a sac or cyst distended with fluid.	Subdural hygroma.
HYPER-HIDROSIS	hyper = overmuch; hidros = sweat; osis = condition	Profuse sweating.	Hyperhidrosis of palms of hands.
HYPER-TROPHY	hyper = overmuch, or excess of; trophe = nourishment	Overgrown or enlarged (not simply swollen).	Hypertrophy of liver may occur in cancer.
ICTERUS	icterus = a yellow bird	A word used to indicate jaundice.	Icterus neonatorum is a jaundiced condition of the newborn.
IDIOPATHIC	idios = one's self; pathos = disease	A term used to show that a disease is self-originated; usually it is thought of as being of unknown cause, and only the functional reaction can be noted.	Idiopathic ulcerative colitis — a severe ulcerative disease of the colon, cause undetermined.

Word	Analysis	Meaning	Example of Use
INCONTI-NENCE	in = not; continere = to contain	Not able to control natural drainage.	Incontinence can be of the bowels as well as of urine.
INCUBATION PERIOD	in = in; cubare = to lie in	The period between contact of an infection and when it appears in a diagnosable stage.	The incubation period in measles is from 14 to 21 days.
INFARCT	infarcire = to fill up	A coagulation necrosis resulting from lack of blood supply to any part.	An infarct of the heart muscle, due to occlusion of a coronary artery, frequently results in death.
IN SITU	in = in; situs = place	In the normal place.	Organs in situ.
INSOMNIA	in = not; somnus = sleep	Inability to sleep.	Insomnia may be caused by worry.
INTROITUS	intro = within; ire = to go	An aperture or entrance.	Vaginal introitus.
JACTITA-TION	jactitare = to toss	A patient tossing about in acute disease.	Jactitation is marked in delirium.

Word	Analysis	Meaning	Example of Use
JAUNDICE	*jaune* = yellow	Yellowness of skin and mucous linings due to absorption of bile into the blood stream.	On examination, the "whites" of the eyes may appear jaundiced.
KALIEMIA	*kali* = potash; *haima* = blood	Having potassium in the blood.	Normal "kaliemia" is 20 milligrams per 100 cc. A wasting disease may cause hypokaliemia.
KELOID	*kelis* = spot, scar; *oid* = form	Dense new tissue growth of skin.	Keloids are found on skin following irritations and injuries.
KERNIG'S SIGN	Vladimir Kernig was a Russian neurologist.	Kernig's sign is positive if by bending the thigh over the abdomen and extending the leg, the motion produces resistance in the leg and pain in the back. Dr. Kernig first used this test.	Kernig's sign may be present in meningitis.
KINESI-THERAPY	*kinesis* = motion; *therapy* = cure	Treatment by exercise.	Kinesitherapy is recommended as a postpartum health measure.

Word	Analysis	Meaning	Example of Use
KRAUROSIS (kraw-ro′sis)	*krauros* = dry; *osis* = state of being	A condition of being dry and shriveled.	This word is usually used in describing a dry condition of the mucous membranes, such as kraurosis of the vulva.
KYPHOSIS	*kyphos* = bent or bowed; *osis* = state of being	A curvature of the spine, humpbacked type.	A child may be born with kyphosis, or it may be the result of infection or injury.
LABIOLOGY	*labium* = lip; *logos* = study of	Lip reading.	Patients with acquired deafness may be interested in labiology.
LAMPRO-PHONIA	*lampros* = clear; *phonê* = voice	Clearness of voice.	Lamprophonia is a quality expected in speaking.
LATENT	*latere* = to lie hidden	Something concealed. (In medicine it is used to express results from infections or diseases which have not manifested themselves over a period of time.)	Latent syphilis.
LEPTO-DERMIC	*leptos* = thin or slender; *derma* = skin	Thin-skinned.	Newborn are considered more leptodermic than adults.

Word	Analysis	Meaning	Example of Use
LESION	*laedere* = to hurt	An injury or disease; any pathology.	A lesion may be a broken bone or an ulcer of the stomach; any morbid structural change.
LETHARGY	*lethargia* = mental slowness or forgetfulness	A condition of drowsiness or slowness of reaction which cannot be overcome by the will.	Types of brain inflammation and overdosage of sedative drugs cause definite lethargy.
LETHO-LOGICA	*lethe* = forgetfulness; *logia* = word	Inability to recall words.	Lethologica frequently occurs as a result of a "little stroke."
LEUKO-DERMA	*leukos* = white; *derma* = skin	White patches of skin.	Acquired leukoderma is more often called vitiligo.
LEUKO-NYCHIA (lu-ko-nik'e-ah)	*leukos* = white; *onyx* = nail; *ia* = condition	White discoloration of nails.	Leukonychia may be a result of fungus invasion.
LIENORENAL	*lien* = spleen; *ren* = kidney	Spleen and kidney.	No masses were felt in the lieno-renal area on examination.
LIGATURE	*ligatura* = a tie	An article used as a thread to tie off a part.	A ligature may be used following removal of a tonsil if bleeding occurs.

Word	Analysis	Meaning	Example of Use
LINEAE ALBI-CANTES	*linea* = line; *albicare* = to be white	White lines.	Lineae albicantes as a result of pregnancy. (White lines on abdomen where skin has been stretched.)
LIPOID	*lipos* = fat; *oid* = like	A thing resembling fat.	"Lipoid" substance or tissue resembles fat tissue but has not been proved to be fat by microchemical methods.*
LIPSOTRI-CHIA	*leipein* = to leave; *trichia* = hair	Falling hair.	Lipsotrichia as a result of infection.
LOCHIA	*lochios* = pertains to childbirth	The discharges following birth of a child.	Foul lochia may indicate infection.
LORDOSIS	*lordos* = bent forward	A type of curvature of spine.	Lordosis occurs in lower spine, giving a swayback appearance.

*This is a necessary "short-cut" statement in routine pathological reports on tissue studies. Microchemical methods to determine the presence of *true* fat are time-consuming and expensive. One must remember that there are other "short cuts" in terminology which are used for similar reasons, and that the adage "a little knowledge is a dangerous thing" applies to the most assiduous student of this book.

Word	Analysis	Meaning	Example of Use
LUES	lues = a plague or spreading disease	The modern meaning is syphilis.	Lues may not be detected in its beginning stage if no outward signs are noticed.
LYCOREXIA (li-ko-reks′-e-ah)	lykos = wolf; orexia = hunger	Wolfish or ravenous appetite.	Lycorexia is more often due to exercise rather than pathology.
LYMPHADE-NOPATHY	lympha = water; aden = gland; pathos = disease	Disease of the lymph glands.	Physical examination may elicit no lymphadenopathy.
MACRO-GNATHIA (mak-ro-na′the-ah)	makros = large; gnathos = jaw	Enlarged jaw.	A congenital macrognathia is often thought to indicate a person with a strong will.
MACULA	macula = a small mark or spot; pl. = maculae	In medicine, it refers to an abnormal spot; a blemish.	Macula of skin or retina of eye.
MALAISE	mal = abnormal or ill; aise = ease	Ill at ease; sick and in distress.	A patient suffering general malaise is sick and uncomfortable all over.

Word	Analysis	Meaning	Example of Use
MALINGERER (mal-in'ger-er)	*malingre* = sickly	One who pretends illness.	A malingerer may have other neuroses.
MARASMUS	*marasmos* = wasting	A gradual wasting of tissues from malnutrition.	Marasmus may occur in infants who cannot retain their feedings.
MEGALO-NYCHOSIS (meg"al-o-nik-o'sis)	*megas* = great; *onyx* = nail; *ia* = condition	Hypertrophy of nails.	Injury to the nail matrix may result in megalonychosis.
MELOMANIA	*melos* = song; *mania* = madness	Obsessive fondness for music.	A characteristic of melomania may produce a great orchestral conductor.
MENARCHE (men-ar'ke)	*mensis* = month; *arche* = beginning	Beginning of menstrual function.	Menarche usually occurs at the age of 12.
MEROPIA	*meros* = part; *opia* = vision	Partial blindness.	Meropia due to glaucoma.

Word	Analysis	Meaning	Example of Use
METABO-LISM	*metabole* = change	The change of nutritive material into substance which is growing and alive.	Basal metabolism is measured by calorie count; so many calories per hour per square meter of body surface.
METASTASIS	*meta* = change; *stasis* = position	Spreading by means of direct invasion or infiltration.	Cancers or malignant diseases go through a process of metastasis.
MICROCORIA	*micros* = small; *corê* = pupil	Small pupil.	Congenital microcoria.
MICRO-GNATHIA	*micros* = small; *gnathos* = jaw	Undue smallness of lower jaw.	Micrognathia is often referred to a chinless person. (One who does not develop a lower jaw.)
MICTURI-TION	*micturire* = to urinate	Urinating.	Infection of the urethra can cause frequent and painful micturition.
MILIARY	*milium* = millet seed	Small and productive or prolific. Miliary in modern use is being applied much in the same fashion as the word metastasis.	A miliary tuberculosis is a quick-spreading type which invades many tissues other than the lungs.

Word	Analysis	Meaning	Example of Use
MONOPHAGIA	monos = single; phagein = to swallow or eat	Craving or eating one kind of food.	Continuous monophagia will result in avitaminosis.
MORBIDITY	morbus = a disease	The quality of being diseased.	Morbidity rate: the ratio of the number of individuals sick (with a particular disease) to a total population.
MORIBUND	moribundus = in a dying state	In a dying condition.	A patient may be moribund.
MORTALITY	mors = death	The quality of being mortal.	Mortality rate: the death rate (usually of a particular condition or disease).
MULTIPA- ROUS	multi = many; parere = to bear	Having given birth to two or more children.	A mother who has borne five children would be described as multiparous, or as a multipara.
MYDRIATIC	mydros = a little hot stone	An agent causing dilatation of the pupil.	Atropine is a mydriatic, as are homatropine, ephedrine.
NANOID	nanus = dwarf; oid = resembling	Dwarfish.	A nanoid condition may be congenital.

Word	Analysis	Meaning	Example of Use
NAUSEA	naus = ship	Shipsickness or seasickness; the ill feeling which comes before vomiting.	The first symptom of many diseases is nausea.
NECROPSY	nekros = dead; opsis = viewing	Examination of a corpse; an autopsy or postmortem examination.	When a person dies without attendance of a physician, the coroner may order a necropsy.
NECROSIS	nekros = dead; osis = condition or process of	Condition or process of tissue dying in a live body.	Necrotic tissue or necrosis may be found in parts of the body where the blood supply to the part has been obstructed.
NEONATAL	neos = new; natus = born	Pertaining to a newborn.	Neonatal deaths occur within 72 hours after a child is born.
NEOPLASM	neos = new; plasma = a thing molded or formed	A new growth; a tumor.	Neoplasms may be either benign or malignant.
NOCTURIA	nox = the night; ouron = urine	Excessive urination at night.	Pressure on the bladder (by a tumor or disease of the kidneys) may cause nocturia.

Word	Analysis	Meaning	Example of Use
NULLIPA-ROUS (nul-ip′a-rus)	nullus = none; parere = to bear	A woman who has never given birth to a child.	A vaginal outlet may be of a nulliparous type.
NYCTALOPIA	nyx = night; alaos = blind; opia = vision	Night blindness.	Persons who suffer nyctalopia should not drive by night.
NYSTAGMUS (nis-tag′mus)	nystagmos = nodding	A quick, uncontrolled movement of the eyeballs. It may be to the side, up and down, rotary or mixed.	One of the symptoms of multiple sclerosis is nystagmus.
OBESE OBESITY	obesus = fat	Excessively fat.	Persons may be judged obese according to certain standards of age and height.
OCCLUSION	occlusus = closed	A part which has been shut off or closed.	A coronary occlusion indicates that the coronary artery has been obstructed, probably by a blood clot. This usually implies an infarction of heart muscle.

Word	Analysis	Meaning	Example of Use
OLIGURIA	oligos = scanty; ouron = urine	Reduced output of urine.	Chronic kidney diseases may produce oliguria.
OMODYNIA	omos = shoulder; odyne = pain	Pain in the shoulder.	Omodynia, a warning of any one of many diseases.
ONCOTHER-APY	onkos = tumor; therapy = treatment	A tumor treatment.	The radiologist prescribes oncotherapy.
ONYCHOMY-COSIS (on"ik-o-mi-ko'sis)	onyx = nail; mykes = fungus; osis = condition	Fungus of the nail.	Monilia is a type of onychomy-cosis. (Tinea unguium is also used to indicate a nail fungus.)
OPHTHALMO-COPIA	ophthalmos = eye; kopos = weariness	Eye fatigue; eyestrain.	Ophthalmocopia may be the result of reading under poor lights.
OPISTHOTIC	opisthen = behind; ous, otos = ear	Situated behind the ear.	Opisthotic pain.
ORIENTA-TION	oriens = arising (used of the sun)	Determination of the position of a person or thing (originally with relation to the rising sun).	Disorientation indicates that one is confused or wandering in mind because he does not know where he is.

Word	Analysis	Meaning	Example of Use
ORONASAL	os, oris = mouth; nasus = nose	Mouth and nose.	Oronasal injection.
ORO-PHARYNX	os, oris = mouth; pharynx = throat	Mouth and throat.	Inflammation of the oropharynx area.
ORTHOPNEA (or-thop-ne'ah)	orthos = straight or upright; pnea = breathing	Being able to breathe only in an upright position.	Cardiac patients frequently suffer from orthopnea and must be propped up in bed.
ORTHO-STATIC	orthos = upright or straight; stasis = standing	Pertaining to or caused by standing upright.	Orthostatic albuminuria is not present during a period of rest in bed.
OSSICLE	os = bone; cle = a diminutive	Small bony structures.	The small bones of the ear; the incus, malleus and stapes are ossicles.
OTOMYCOSIS	ous, otos = ear; mykes = fungus; osis = condition	Fungus of the ear.	Aspergillus is a frequently found otomycosis.
OTORRHEA	ous, otos = ear; rrhea = flow	A draining ear.	Infections of the ear usually are accompanied by otorrhea.

Word	Analysis	Meaning	Example of Use
PACHY-GLOSSIA (pak-e-glos'-e-ah)	*pachys* = thick; *glossa* = tongue; *ia* = condition	Thick tongue (or perhaps hyperglossia).	Pachyglossia will make feeding of infants a problem.
PALLIATIVE	*palliare* = to hide or cloak	In medicine it means to give relief by treatment but not necessarily to cure.	Crushing the phrenic nerve is often a palliative procedure, having a temporary effect of putting one lung "at rest."
PALPATION	*palpare* = to feel	Touching with the fingers the external surfaces of the body in order to feel the structures beneath.	Palpation of the neck will detect enlarged glands.
PALPITA-TION	*palpitare* = to throb or quiver	A fluttering condition.	Palpitation of the heart (usually felt by the patient).
PANNUS	*pannus* = cloth or web	A covering, full of small vessels, which may be seen over the cornea of the eye.	A pannus due to infection or allergy.
PAPULE	*papula* = a pimple; pl. = *papulae*	The term refers to a small swelling not containing fluid or pus.	Skin may be covered with papulae.

Word	Analysis	Meaning	Example of Use
PARESTHE-SIA	*para* = beside (normal) ; *esthesis* = sensation	A burning, prickling or feeling of numbness.	Having the foot "go to sleep" is a form of paresthesia.
PAROXYSM	*para* = beside or beyond; *oxys* = sharp	A seizure beyond control.	A paroxysm of coughing.
PARTURI-TION	*parturire* = to be in labor	Giving birth to a child.	Left occipito-anterior is the most frequent type of parturition.
PENTA-DACTYL (pen-tah-dak'til)	*penta* = five; *dactyl* = finger	Five fingers.	A pentadactyl count is normal for one hand.
PERCUSSION	*percussio* = a striking	A method of diagnosis done by tapping over parts of the body to distinguish areas of dullness, density or hollowness.	Percussion over the border of the liver is done to show its size or position.
PERISTAL-SIS (per-is-tal'sis)	*peri* = around; *stalsis* = contraction	The waves or movements of the intestines which propel its contents.	Peristalsis begins as soon as food enters the tract.

Word	Analysis	Meaning	Example of Use
PETECHIA (pe-te'ke-ah)	petechia = a small spot; pl. = petechiae	Small areas of hemorrhage under the skin or in an organ.	Petechiae are a sign of purpura.
PICA	pica = magpie	A craving for unnatural foods; depraved appetite for foods.	Pica is a craving for strange foods during pregnancy.
PNEUMOCO-NIOSIS (nu"mo-ko-ne-o'sis)	pneumon = lung; conis = dust; osis = condition	Inhalation of small particles into lung.	Silicosis is a form of pneumoconiosis.
POLYPNEA (pol-ip-ne'ah)	poly = many; pnoia = respiration	Increased respiratory rate.	Polypnea is usually present with fever.
POLYPUS	poly = many; pous = foot; pl. = polypi	Smooth growths on mucous linings.	Polypi are the result of enlargement of mucous membrane.
POLYURIA	poly = much; ouron = urine	Much urine.	Polyuria may be the result of an increased fluid intake.
PRE-CORDIAL	pre = before; cor = heart	Referring to the region overlying the heart.	A precordial pain.

Word	Analysis	Meaning	Example of Use
PRENATAL	pre = before; natus = birth	During pregnancy or before the birth of a child.	Disturbances arising during pregnancy are prenatal diseases, as they refer to the infant.
PRESBYOPIA (pres-be-o'pe-ah)	presbys = old; opia = vision	Loss of accommodation in vision from near to distant points.	Presbyopia occurs in most persons after the age of 40.
PRIMIPARA	primus = first; parere = to bear	A woman who has given birth to a first child.	The word "primipara" may be found in the pregnancy history of a patient.
PROGERIA	pro = before; geras = old age	A child who takes on the appearance of old age.	Progeria may be diagnosed in the infancy or adolescent ages.
PROGNOSIS	pro = before; gnosis = knowledge	Foretelling possible outcome of a disease.	Prognosis is for recovery, improvement or unimprovement of a patient.
PROSTHESIS	pros = to; thesis = putting	Replacement of a missing part by an artificial substitute.	Eye prosthesis.
PROTOPLASM	protos = first; plasma = tissue	First tissue formed in a living cell.	Functional protoplasm.

Word	Analysis	Meaning	Example of Use
PRURITUS (pru-ri′tus)	*prurire* = to itch	Intense itching.	Pruritus may be of the skin as a whole or localized.
PTOSIS (to′sis)	*ptosis* = fall	An organ dropping down out of its normal place.	Ptosis of abdominal organs is called splanchnoptosis; of the kidney, nephroptosis.
PUER-PERIUM (pu-er-pe′re-um)	*puer* = child; *parere* = to bring forth	The lying-in period after child-birth. It covers the period from birth of the child until return to normal of the uterus.	During the puerperium, the mother is checked carefully to note any signs of hemorrhage.
PULSE	*pulsare* = to strike or beat; *pulsus* = stroke	Expansion and contraction of an artery which can be felt by the finger.	Pulse rate is a method of record-ing the normal heart rate.
PURULENT	*pus* = pus	Consisting of or containing pus.	An infected wound may become purulent.
PYOMETRIUM	*pyon* = pus; *metra* = uterus	Pus within the uterus.	Pyometrium due to streptococcus.
PYOPTYSIS (pi-op′tis-is)	*pyon* = pus; *ptysis* = spitting	Expectoration of pus.	Pyoptysis due to oral abscess.

Word	Analysis	Meaning	Example of Use
PYREXIA	*pyr* = fire; *exia* = condition	Condition of being feverish.	Pyrexia is a first symptom of many diseases.
QUIESCENT	*quiescere* = to be at rest	A word used to express inactivity of a disease.	Tuberculosis in a quiescent stage.
RACHIALGIA (ra-ke-al'je-ah)	*rachis* = spine or vertebral column; *algos* = pain	Pain in vertebral column.	Rachialgia (neuralgia) would require investigation to determine cause.
RADICULITIS	*radix* = root (radicula is diminutive); *itis* = inflammation	Inflammation of nerve root.	Radiculitis may be the cause of rachialgia.
RÂLE	*râle* = rattle	A rattle-like sound.	Chest râles.
REFLEX	*reflectere* = to turn back	Involuntary action or reaction.	Reflex pain; postural reflex.
REGURGI-TATION	*re* = again; *gurgitare* = to gush	A flowing or gushing backward.	Regurgitation of food with belching.
RHINOPHYMA	*rhis* = nose; *phyma* = growth or swelling	Nodular swelling and congestion of nose.	Rhinophyma is the result of dilation of capillaries.

Word	Analysis	Meaning	Example of Use
RHONCHUS	*rhonchos* = a snore; pl. = *rhonchi*	A coarse sound which resembles a snore.	Rhonchus of the chest or throat.
RIGOR	*rigor* = stiffness, cold	Chill or cold shiver.	Malarial rigor.
ROMBERG'S SIGN	Moritz Heinrich Romberg, a German neurologist.	A swaying of the body when a patient stands with his feet close together and his eyes closed.	Romberg's sign may be present in neurosyphilis.
SCOTOMA	*skotos* = darkness or gloom; pl. = *scotomata*	A blind spot in the visual field of the eye.	A positive scotoma is one in which the patient sees a dark spot.
SEBORRHEA	*sebum* = suet or grease; *rhoia* = a flow	Excessive discharge from sebaceous glands of skin; excessive oiliness of skin.	Many reactions occur as a result of seborrhea, e.g., seborrhea of scalp.
SEDATION	*sedare* = to settle or calm down	An agent used to allay excitement.	A patient under sedation may sleep peacefully.
SENILE	*senilis* = old	Pertaining to old age.	Senile psychosis.
SEPSIS	*sepsis* = decay or infection	An infection or poisoning.	Puerperal sepsis.

Word	Analysis	Meaning	Example of Use
SEQUELA	*sequela* = follower pl. = *sequelae*	A morbid condition as a result of disease.	A patient may have several childhood diseases without sequelae.
SIALOLITH (si-al'o-lith)	*sialon* = saliva; *lithos* = stone	Calculus in the salivary duct.	Submaxillary sialolith.
SIBLING	diminutive of *sib* = a little blood relation	Children of the same generation. (Brothers and sisters.)	It may be stated in the family history that there are three siblings, all living and well.
SIDEROPENIA	*sideros* = iron; *penia* = poverty	Iron deficiency in the blood.	Sideropenia may be the cause of anemia.
SINGULTUS	*singultus* = sob	A hiccough.	Singultus of a "nervous" stomach.
SOMNAMBU-LISM	*somnus* = sleep; *ambulare* = to walk about	Sleepwalking.	
SPASMODIC	*spasmos* = drawing tight	Like a spasm; characterized by a sudden tightening.	Spasmodic seizures of the muscle.
SPASTIC	*spastikos* = of the nature of a spasm	Characterized by a drawing or stiffening of muscles.	Spastic movements are stiff and awkward.

Word	Analysis	Meaning	Example of Use
SPUTUM	*spuere* = to spit or spew	Spittle.	Sputum examination is essential when tuberculosis is suspected.
STEATOPYGIA (ste"at-o-pij'e-ah)	*steatos* = fat; *pyge* = rump or buttocks	Excessive fatness of the buttocks.	Steatopygia is an unbecoming characteristic.
STENOSIS	*stenos* = narrow; *osis* = a condition of	A narrowing or closing of a part.	Pyloric stenosis.
STERNUTA-TION	*sternutatio* = sneezing	Act of sneezing.	Successive sternutations may mean an allergic condition or an oncoming cold.
STRANGURY (strang'u-re)	*stranx* = strangulation; *ouron* = urine	Painful urination, drop by drop.	Spasm of the urinary bladder will cause strangury.
STRIA	*stria* = a streak, line or furrow; pl. = *striae*	Lines formed by habit or conditions.	Striae atrophicae, following pregnancy or reduction of fat.
STRIDOR	*stridere* = to make a creaking sound	A harsh whistling sound.	Stridor, following inhalation of a foreign body.

Word	Analysis	Meaning	Example of Use
SUCCUSSION	*succutere* = to shake up	Shaking or turning of a patient to detect the presence of fluid in a cavity.	Succussion in the diagnosis of hydropneumothorax.
SUPPRES-SION	*suppressio* = holding back	A sudden cessation of secretion.	Urinary suppression (by the kidney), as distinct from retention in the bladder.
SYMBLEPH-ARON (sim-blef'ar-on)	*syn* = together; *blepharon* = eyelid	Adhesion of lids to the eyeball.	Total, anterior or posterior symblepharon may be congenital.
SYNCOPE (sin'ko-pe)	*syn* = with; *koptein* = to strike, crush	Fainting.	Syncope may follow an emotional shock.
SYNDROME	*syn* = together; *dromos* = a running	A set of symptoms which occur together.	Ménière's syndrome (severe vertigo with nausea and vomiting).
TABACOSIS	*tabacum* = tobacco; *osis* = condition	Inhalation of tobacco dust.	Tabacosis is sometimes found in those who work in tobacco factories.

Word	Analysis	Meaning	Example of Use
TACHY-PHAGIA (tak-e-fa'-je-ah)	*tachis* = rapid; *phagein* = to swallow or eat	Rapid eating.	Mastication is mostly incomplete in those who practice tachyphagia.
TACHYPNEA (tak-ip-ne'ah)	*tachis* = fast; *pnea* = breathing	Rapid breathing. (Not dyspnea, difficult or labored breathing.)	Tachypnea on exertion.
TACTILE	*tactilis* = touchable	Perceptible to touch, a basic sensation.	Tactile fremitus; tactile sensation.
TENESMUS	*teinesmos* = a straining	Painful or ineffectual attempts to evacuate the bowels or urinary bladder.	Tenesmus with acute diarrhea.
TETRA-PLEGIA	*tetra* = four; *plege* = stroke	Paralysis of all four extremities.	Tetraplegia and quadriplegia are synonymous terms. Trauma to the spinal cord could cause paralysis of all four extremities.
THERAPY THERAPEU-TICS	*therapeuein* = to serve or take care of	The art or science of healing.	Drug therapy, physical therapy, or psychotherapy, for the immediate needs of the patient.

Word	Analysis	Meaning	Example of Use
THERMO-PLEGIA	*therme* = heat; *plege* = stroke	Heatstroke or sunstroke.	Elderly persons seem to suffer thermoplegia more often than others.
THRILLS	*thrill* = a tremor or vibration	Reaction felt on application of hand or finger tips to body.	Systolic thrills (vibration with cardiac systole).
THROMBUS	*thrombos* = a lump	A plug or clot of blood in a vessel or heart cavity which remains stationary.	Coronary thrombus (may lead to infarction).
TIC	*tic* = twitching	A twiching movement which may be due to habit or pain, or be involuntary.	Tic of facial muscles (a manifestation of hysteria).
TINNITUS	*tinnitus* = a tinkling	A ringing or metallic sound.	Tinnitus of ears.
TOXIC	*toxon* = a bow (poison for arrows was called *toxikon* whence *pharmakon*, whence *toxikon* acquired the meaning of "poisonous")	In the state of being poisoned or absorbing poisons.	A toxic condition of pregnancy. (Not necessarily a known toxin such as that of diphtheria or botulism.)

Word	Analysis	Meaning	Example of Use
TRANSIL-LUMINATE	*trans* = through; *illuminare* = to light	To pass a strong light through to an interior cavity, usually for diagnostic reasons.	To transilluminate the paranasal sinuses.
TRAUMA	*trauma* = a wound; pl. = *traumata*	An injury or wound.	Trauma due to birth or accident.
TREMOR	*tremere* = to shake	A trembling.	Tremor of a muscle.
TRICHOR-RHEA	*tricos* = hair; *rhoia* = a flow	Rapid loss of hair.	Trichorrhea may be caused by having high fever.
TRISMUS	*trizein* = to gnash	A word used to indicate lockjaw because of the grinding of teeth.	Trismus or tetanus.
TROPHE-DEMA	*trophe* = nourish-ment; *oidema* = swelling	More or less permanent swelling of feet and legs.	Trophedema with ascites.
TUBERCULE	*tuber* = a knob; *culus* = diminutive	A small nodule or rounded eminence.	Bone tubercule. (Not necessarily tuberculosis, which received its name, as a disease, from its propensity to form these lesions.)

Word	Analysis	Meaning	Example of Use
TUMOR	*tumere* = to swell	A mass or swelling which serves no useful purpose; a neoplasm; a new growth.	Benign or malignant tumors.
TUSSIS	*tussis* = cough	Cough.	Tussis convulsiva or pertussis is whooping cough.
ULCER	*ulcus* = ulcer	A sore; necrosis; loss of substance.	Duodenal ulcer.
VACCINE	*vacca* = cow	Originally this term was used to mean injection of cowpox virus to produce an immunity from smallpox. It has come to mean the hypodermic injection of any preparation of attenuated or killed bacteria or viruses, in order to produce an immunity.	Allergy vaccines; pertussis vaccine.
VARIX	*varix* = a dilated vein	Varicose vein; also varicose condition.	Varix of saphenous vein.
VASOSPASM	*vas* = vessel; *spasmos* = contraction or tightening	Constricting of a blood vessel.	Vasospasm of leg.

Word	Analysis	Meaning	Example of Use
VENTILA-TION	*ventilare* = to wave in air, to fan	To give vent to one's feelings; to open up and tell all.	Some neuroses are aided by ventilation.
VENTRAL	*venter* = belly	Pertaining to the belly side; abdominal.	Ventral hernia.
VENTRICLE	*ventriculus* = small cavity	Any small cavity.	Ventricles of the heart or brain.
VERMIFORM	*vermis* = worm; *forma* = shape	Wormlike.	Vermiform appendix.
VERRUCA	*verruca* = a wart	A wart.	Verruca plana.
VERSION	*vertere* = to turn	The obstetrical procedure of turning the fetus in utero.	Version and extraction of a baby.
VESTIGIAL	*vestigium* = a footprint	Rudimentary parts; remains or traces of.	Vestigial remnants sometimes are the basis of tumorlike growths.
VIRUS	*virus* = a poison	Extremely poisonous or infectious agent.	The virus of smallpox.
VOIDING	*void* = to cast out waste	The act of urinating or defecating.	The patient's hours of voiding as recorded on a chart.

Word	Analysis	Meaning	Example of Use
WHEAL	wale or weal = mark made by a whip, or a raised ridge	A raised skin defect, usually pustular.	The wheal is the primary lesion in urticaria.
XANTHOMA (zan-tho'-mah)	xanthos = yellow; oma = tumor	Deposits of lipoids in the skin which are characterized by flat plaques of yellow color.	Xanthoma due to metabolism.
XERODERMA (ze-ro-der'-mah)	xeros = dry; derma = skin	Dry, rough skin.	Xeroderma with a scaly desquamation.
XEROSIS	xeros = dry; osis = condition	Condition of dryness.	Xerosis of skin.
XIPHOID	xiphos = sword; oid = like	Swordlike.	Xiphoid process (a cartilage below the sternum, often used as a descriptive landmark).
ZOSTER	zoster = girdle	Formed around or encircling; in medicine it means "shingles" (an acute inflammatory disease consisting of grouped vesicles following the course of cutaneous nerves).	Herpes zoster.

SAMPLE EXERCISE NO. I

Word	Analysis	Meaning	Example of Use
1. PSYCHONEUROSIS			
2. TYPHOID			
3. TORTICOLLIS			
4. THERMOMETER			
5. TALIPES EQUINO-VALGUS			
6. TELEPATHY			
7. SUBACUTE			
8. PILONIDAL			
9. OTOSCLEROSIS			
10. SEPTICEMIA			
11.			
12.			
13.			
14.			
15.			
16.			
17.			
18.			
19.			
20.			

SAMPLE EXERCISE NO. II

Diagnosis	Definition	Name of Service or Services on which usually treated	Name of Operation (if operable)
1. Abscess of arm			
2. Eczema			
3. Blepharitis			
4. Hallux valgus			
5. Coronary thrombosis			
6. Cicatrix of skin due to burns			
7. Cholelithiasis			
8. Stricture of urethra			
9. Parturition			
10. Mastoiditis			

PART II

THE MEDICAL RECORD

Introduction

Beginners in any service of the medical field should be familiar with the medical record and its values. It serves the patient primarily, but has many values to the physician and to hospital administration. It serves the patient in his present and future illnesses. It is a storehouse of knowledge for the physician and hospital since, in it, the physician may read all recordings of his medical findings and the hospital may justify its existence in having proof that it has served the community and has given good care to the sick.

Accrediting boards state that the medical record is the criterion for evaluating service to the patient. Accreditations or rating of a school of medicine, a hospital, clinics and various training programs within any medical center depend much upon the excellence of medical records. The number of trainees permitted in any one of the medical or paramedical programs is determined by the number of patients and the types of experiences (diseases, operations, examinations and treatments) to which a trainee is exposed. Training levels are also determined by these related experiences. Therefore, medical records must be concordantly perfect to enable accreditation inspectors to make proper decisions and give just ratings. Patients, physicians, trainees and the medical centers alike may be benefited.

Related experiences, through careful studies of medical records, are of value to education and medical research. The results of these studies find their way into publications and make up the priceless contributions to medical libraries. These studies advance medical science around the world.

A patient is not to be referred to as a "case." An instance of injury or a history of disease may be referred to as a case and is of value in statistical studies and clinical reports. A physician does not treat a case. The physician deals with human beings in one of the most dignified personal relationships, that of physician to patient, and a medical record which shows that a physician has assumed full responsibility in this relationship, will be a good record.

No history or physical examination can ever be regarded as truly complete. From the diagnostic point of view, a specialist is a physician who can secure a better history and do a more complete physical examination because of his greater experience in a particular field of medicine. A history which has clinical value is usually not given freely by a patient, nor can it be extracted by an untrained individual. It must be obtained by an interviewer who is: (1) knowledgeable in patterns of disturbed physiology; (2) careful to describe his findings in accurate and clear wording; and (3) conscientious in securing and recording the patient's description of complaints and illnesses. This type of interviewer writes a good history because he knows the questions to ask. Each particular disclosure may suggest several disease entities to him. He knows the history relevant to the different possibilities and the effective way in which his inquiry must be made. Important information obtained in this manner could never be procured if the physician relied solely on the history volunteered by the patient.

The physical examination is pursued with the greatest care and energy also, especially in the areas where the patient's history and the examiner's experience indicate that results are apt to be most fruitful.

In both the history and physical examination there are certain minimum requirements. They will be noted in the ensuing outlines. Positive findings in the individual patient will determine where the minimum should be expanded.

It must also be noted that the history and physical examination alone cannot make a good medical record, nor can laboratory work, tests and treatment techniques be carried out alone by the clinician. It takes the combined efforts and recorded findings of medically and paramedically trained persons who explore and determine specific examinations and treatments which have been suggested as necessary to understand an individual ailment.

COMPOSITION OF MEDICAL RECORD

(Write Clearly. Use Only Approved Abbreviations.)

IDENTIFICATION

Identification must be sufficient to set apart clearly each patient's individual medical record. Since these data are sometimes used to fill in birth and death certificates, sufficient identification must be obtained for these purposes. The minimum information necessary includes: Full name (surname, first name and middle names) ; Address; Date of birth; Age; Race; Sex; Mother's maiden name; and Father's full name.

The examiner should make sure to check the accuracy of the spelling of names. On readmissions the address must be brought up to date. The examiner might also note that the age is correctly recorded.

Mention and be specific about referring physician or agency if patient did not come primarily of his own accord. Reports must be sent to the referee later.

MEDICAL HISTORY

CHIEF COMPLAINT

This is a brief statement, written as far as possible in the patient's own words, giving his reason for seeking medical care and duration of symptoms. Examples: "Fainting spells." "Stomach trouble for five years." "Sore side for three days."

PRESENT ILLNESS (write in past tense)

Present illness covers the onset of first symptoms of the disease, its location, duration, frequency of occurrence and severity. The patient will use many non-medical terms to express himself, but the physician will write them in medical language.

Examples: anorexia, eructation, vertigo, dyspnea, polyuria, edema of extremities.

The writer should organize the present illness with care. It should include all pertinent positive and negative information. When the present illness involves several systems, the development of symptoms in each system should be described in separate paragraphs which are chronologically organized. Symptoms should be fully and accurately described but not interpreted into diagnoses by the interviewer.

Previous treatment of the current illness should be noted in detail, giving names of physicians and hospitals involved in the care.

ALLERGIC TENDENCIES

Sensitivity to items experienced in daily living are of major importance. Inquire specifically about food sensitivities. Ask about known reactions to drugs or other agents (tetanus antitoxin — T.A.T., penicillin, local administration of anesthesia in dental work or pain medicines). Note episodes of eczema, urticaria, allergic rhinitis or asthma. On the medical record enter remarks on the positive findings in this category so clearly that they may be easily recognized by all persons caring for the patient.

PAST HISTORY

The past history will include items apparently not relevant to the present illness.

1. Patient's estimate of general health. Childhood diseases (measles, epidemic parotitis and pertussis, chickenpox) and statement of immunizations.

2. Significant data from past physical examinations (school, military service, industrial, insurance or visits to other physicians).

3. Previous hospital admissions, major operations, injuries and past serious illnesses should be noted. Summaries of other hospital admissions should be reviewed if possible and the positive findings recorded.

4. Weight: Recent change and why — voluntary or involuntary — minimum adult weight, maximum adult weight, present weight.

5. Review of systems: A full description of positive findings should be written. (Note: Examples of the medical language used to describe findings are listed below under each system or specific organ. However, the inquiry is made in terms that the patient will understand.)

Skin: Eruption. Pigmentation. Birthmarks. Bruisings. Pruritus.

Bones, Joints, Muscles: Past fractures. Change in posture. Pain. Tenderness. Swelling. Limitation of motion. Overlying redness. Muscle spasms and where. Limp or weakness of arms or legs.

Head: Cephalalgia (dull, throbbing, location, periodicity, duration).

Eyes: Pain. Inflammation. Diplopia. Vision (wears glasses).

Ears: Ache. Drainage. Hearing. Tinnitus.

Nose and Throat: Epistaxis. Sinusitis. Colds. Frequent sore throat. Rhinorrhea. Spasmodic attacks of sneezing. Postnasal drip. Olfactory sense.

Breast: Pain. Masses. Drainage.

Cardiorespiratory: General exercise tolerance. Dyspnea. Wheezing. Cough. Sputum. Hemoptysis. Chest pain, including character and precipitating events. Palpitation. Edema. Syncope.

Gastrointestinal: Appetite. Ageusia. Teeth. Buccal and lingual lesions. Dysphagia. Aerophagia. Geophagia. Abdominal pain or discomfort. Distention. Borborygmus. Nausea. Vomiting. Hematemesis. Jaundice. Changes in bowel habits. Constipation. Diarrhea. Stool color (normal, clay, hematochezia, tarry).   Rectal pain, pruritus or bleeding.   Laxatives.

Genitourinary: Retention of urine. Frequency. Stream force. Tenesmus. Incontinence. Enuresis. Nocturia. Polyuria. Dysuria. Hematuria. Renal colic. Stones. Urethral or vaginal discharge. Noticeable lesions. Impotence.

Menstrual: Age at first period.   Last menstrual period. Duration in days.   Interval in days.   Regularity.   Flow (scanty, moderate, excessive).   Amenorrhea.   Dysmenorrhea.   Associated symptoms.   Metrorrhagia.   Odor.

Venereal: Lues. Gonorrhea. Lymphogranuloma. Inguinal granuloma.   Chancroid.   Previous S.T.S.   Previous treatment.   Spinal fluid examinations.

Neuropsychiatric: Neurogenic weakness (local or generalized). Spasticity. Tremor. Tic. Vertigo. Unsteadiness of gait.   Tingling.   Paresthesia or complete numbness. Loss of consciousness. Convulsions. Sleep pattern. Drug habits.   Defective memory.   Lack of concentration or coordination.   Special fears (phobias) or preoccupation. Lethargy.

FAMILY HISTORY

This part of the history should list the patient's parents and siblings, making note of the current status of each. Example: Father, age 62, living and well;   mother, died at age of 40 of pneumonia;   one brother age 24, living and well;   two sisters, one died in infancy, cause unknown, one age 18, living and well.

The family history should also include a specific statement regarding the presence or absence of any of the diseases showing hereditary traits. Examples are diabetes, hypertension, heart disease, kidney disease, tuberculosis, malignancies, neurological and mental diseases, epilepsy, allergies, bleeding diseases or diseases similar to present illness.

MARITAL HISTORY

The marital history relates to age at time of marriage: Duration of marriage.   Age and health of mate.   Pregnancies. Living children (ages and state of health).

PERSONAL HISTORY

The personal history is mainly to define the personality and emotional traits of the patient. Attempt to bring out and distinguish personal characteristics.   Dominant moods.   Stability.   Reaction to stress, to present illness and environment and to examiner.   Obtain history of emotional relation to parents and family. This is often significant and helpful. Examiner should note his opinion of reliability of the history.

SOCIAL HISTORY

The social part of the history covers the patient's habits from both a social and occupational standpoint and its possible relationship to the present illness.   Note occupation.   Ability to work after previous illnesses.   Home conditions.   Family and financial worries.   Habits (relaxation, eating habits and dietary adequacy, use of tobacco, coffee, tea and alcohol).

PHYSICAL EXAMINATION

(Write in Present Tense)

The physical examination, except where emergency treatment is given for minor injuries, covers the whole of the body and is written in sequence by regions and anatomical systems. Abnormalities, even the most obvious ones, will not be found unless the examiner specifically looks for them. The terms listed below, under each anatomical region or system, are those frequently used to add to the picture of that area. The medical language is inexhaustible and the terms used in each pattern are by no means all-inclusive. They must be supplemented wherever required by the findings of the examining physician. Diagrams should be drawn wherever possible to supplement the physical picture.

First to be noted is the temperature, pulse, respiration, height, weight and blood pressure (sitting and supine). In hypertensive patients the blood pressure should be taken of both arms and legs.

GENERAL STATEMENT

The general statement covers a description of the patient as observed by the physician when he begins the examination. Apparent age (agerasia, progeria). Body nutrition. Position (supine, prone, sitting). Apparent degree of illness. Facial expression of discomfort. Obvious abnormalities. Body odors. Example: The patient is a pleasant, white, obese, male, lying comfortably in bed, who appears to be his stated age of 50; or, the patient is a white male of about 50 years of age who appears to be in pain and is restlessly tossing about in bed.

SKIN

Color. Temperature by touch. Texture (soft, glabrous, pachydermatous, dermatolysis). Moisture. Eruptions: nature (macular, papular, florescent, desquamating), distribution, configuration. Pigmentation. Petechiae. Telangiectasia. Atheroma. Nodules. Trophic changes. Secondary infections. Cicatrix. Flushing. Verrucae. Nevi.

HAIR

Color. Texture. Distribution (hirsute, alopecia).

LYMPH NODES

External examination of occipital, cervical, supraclavicular, axillary, epitrochlear and inguinal groups. Size. Hardness. Tenderness. Mobility. Suppuration.

HEAD

Skull: general contour, sutures, fontanelles. Scalp: lesions, tenderness, contusions, lacerations, scars.

EARS

Shape. Hearing ability. Otorrhea. Cerumen. Tympanic membrane. Mastoid tenderness. Auricular tophi.

EYES

Lids: edema, blepharitis, ptosis, entropion, ectropion, symblepharon, chalazion, cilia. Expression. Color. Conjunctiva: pale, injected. Sclera: injection, color. Ocular tension. Corneal scars and opacities. Cataracts. Rough visual acuity. Exophthalmos. Enophthalmos. Extra-ocular movements. Strabismus. Nystagmus. Scotomata. Pupils: equality, size, shape, reaction to light and accommodation. Ophthalmoscopic examination: disc, vessels, fundus, macula. Brows.

FACE

Symmetry. Weakness. Movements or tics. Pain or burning sensation. Edema. Flushing. Cicatricial areas. Bony structures.

NOSE AND SINUSES

Nose: Shape. Breathing space. Mucosa. Furuncles. Foreign bodies. Crustings. Ulcerations. Perforations. Drainage. Septal deviations. Obstruction. Epistaxis.

Sinuses: Tenderness. Transillumination to show clear or cloudy spaces. Polyps. Exudation.

MOUTH AND THROAT

Breath: Foul. Acetone. Sweet.

Lips: Color of mucosa. Herpes. Dryness. Harelip.

Buccal surface: Ulcers. Eruptions. Stomatitis. White patchy areas. Fistulae. Cysts.

Tongue: Color. Coating. Dry or moist. Fissures or geographic tracings. Papillae. Trichoglossia. Macroglossia. Lingual tonsils. Protrusion. Tremor. Deviation. Ankyloglossia.

Salivary and sublingual glands: Sialadenitis. Ptyalism. Calculus. Ranula.

Palate: Arch (breadth and elongation). Perforation. Clefts. Lesions. Torus.

Teeth: Type. Orthodontic order. Number present (adentia). Reparable condition. Full or partial dentures. Deciduous or permanent. Rakelike. Notched. Loose. General hygiene. Caries.

Gums: Gingivitis. Swelling. Ulceration. Bleeding. Parulis. Alveolar status. Pyorrhea.

Pharynx: Color (reddened or white patches). Faucial pillars. Tonsils (present, removed, tags, regrowth, exudate, hypertrophied). Spasms. Dysphagia. Branchial cleft or vestige. Gag reflex.

Uvula: Injected. Elongated or shortened. Paralysis.

Larynx: Inflammation. Edema. Stridor. Voice: Hoarseness, aphonia, dysphonia, eunuchoid, changing voice in puberty.

NECK

Shape. Muscles. Mobility. Torticollis. Venous distention. Pulsations. Thyroid palpability. Bruits over vessels as well as thyroid should be sought. Position of trachea in episternal notch. Tracheal tug. Lymphadenopathy (submaxillary, anterior and posterior cervicals and general lymph nodes).

BREASTS

Type. Development. Gynecomastia. Secretions. Tenderness. Condition in relation to menstrual interval. Masses (palpate in several positions). Scars. Varicosities. Lactating. Galactorrhea. Nipples (supernumerary, thelitis, fissures, inversion).

THORAX

Shape: Funnel chest. Pigeon breast. Flail chest. Barrel chest without emphysema.

Symmetry. Motion on each side. Retraction of interspaces. Ostensible respiratory phenomena. Emphysematous. Precordial bulge. Bony prominences and deformities. Subcostal angle.   Tender costosternal or other joints.   Position of scapula.   Scars.   Sinuses.   *Measure chest expansion.*

LUNGS

Expansion.   Pain on respiration.   Retraction.   Lag.   Peripheral circulation cyanosis.

Rate and type of breathing: Tachypnea.   Bradypnea. Rhythm.   Depth.   Thoracic.   Abdominal.   Dyspnea.   Orthopnea.   Apnea.   Periodic breathing.

Palpation: Tactile fremitus (increased, decreased, normal). Friction rub.

Percussion: Resonance.   Hyperresonance or decreased. Dullness.   Flatness.   Levels and excursions of diaphragm bilaterally.

Auscultation: Breath sounds increased or decreased.   Bronchial.   Bronchovesicular.   Tubular.   Cavernous.   Metallic. Bronchophony.   Egophony.   Rales: moist,   dry,   medium, fine,   coarse.   Friction rubs.

Show position of mediastinum and trachea.

HEART

Precordial impulse: Character.   Location by palpation and inspection.   Shocks.   Thrills.

Percussion: Borders: base (interspace),   apex (interspace and cm. from midsternal and midclavicular lines),   left border (distance in cm. from midsternal and midclavicular lines at level of maximal impulse),   right border.

Diagram above to show borders.

Auscultation: Rate (bradycardia, tachycardia).   Rhythm. Heart tones.   Gallops.   Murmurs: Location, time in cardiac cycle, quality, intensity (grade i to vi), transmission. (Listen in left lateral and sitting positions.)   Friction rubs. A_2 and P_2.

Blood vessels and pulses: Arterial walls (sclerosis, dilatations, aneurysms, enlargement. Radial pulses (quality, rate, rhythm, force). Capillary pulse. Venous pulse. Abnormal vascular structures. Presence of dorsalis pedis and posterior tibial pulses.

ABDOMEN

Type: Scaphoid. Flat. Rounded. Protuberant. *Scars:* Diagram — . Umbilicus. Herniae. Diastasis recti. Pulsations. Visible peristalsis. Tenderness. Rebound tenderness. Spasms. Borborygmus. Tympany. Masses (location, size, form, movable, consistency). Succussion sound. Ascites. Placement of internal organs by palpation, percussion and auscultation.

Liver: Borders of dullness. If palpable — cm. below costal margin. Edge (rounded, sharp, irregularities). Bruits. Rubs.

Spleen: Borders of dullness. If palpable — dimensions, irregularities, notching, friction rubs.

Kidneys: Palpability. Mobility. Size. Costovertebral angle tenderness.

RECTUM

Sphincter. Eruption. Hemorrhoids. Fissures. Fistulae. Prolapse. Polyps.

Prostate: Size. Symmetry. Consistency. Nodules.

Rectal ampulla: Feces. Masses in mucosa. Rectal shelf. Tenderness.

GENITALIA — MALE

Development. Scars. Lesions. Hernial rings. Hydrocele. Varicocele. Prepuce. Urethral orifice (hypospadias, strictures, discharge). Testes. Epididymis.

GENITALIA — FEMALE

Perineum. Condylomata. Introitus. Discharge. *Cervix:* (do routine cancer tests on all over age 35), lacerations, lesions. *Uterus:* Fundus, anteversion, retroversion, retroflexion, size, prolapse.

MUSCULOSKELETAL SYSTEM

Extremities, hands and feet: Nails (unguis incarnatus). Cyanosis. Clubbing of fingers. Joint enlargement. Hallux valgus. Malformations. Polydactylism. Syndactylism. Swelling. Heat. Tenderness. Paresthesia. Atrophy. Callosities. Limitation of movement. Muscle strength (pinch and grip). Plantar and palmar surfaces (nevi, nodules, verruca, sweating). Varicosities. Walking ability.

Bones and joints: General structure. Deformities. Inflammation. Tenderness. Swelling. Pain on motion. Range of motion. Stability. Contracture. Ankylosis (degree). Atrophy. Fluid. Crepitus. Scars. Muscle strength. Flaccid or spastic paralysis.

Spine: (All segments) Flexion. Extension. Rotation. Percussion. Digital palpations. Alignment. Lateral bending. Scoliosis, kyphosis, lordosis. Posture (sitting and standing).

NEUROLOGICAL SURVEY

Gait and associated movements: Limping. Arm movements. Romberg test.

Muscle status: Muscle power (myasthenia, myotonia). Atrophy. Rigidity. Flaccidity. Tics. Tremors. Spasms. Adventitious movements.

Reflexes: Biceps. Triceps. Radial. Tendon. Knee and ankle jerks. Abdominal. Cremasteric. Nerve stretching tests.

Sensory: Vibratory sense in extremities. Touch (position, pain and temperature sense when indicated).

MENTAL STATUS

Attitude. Co-operation. Expression. Euphoria. Depression. Exhilarated or indifferent. Coma. Stuporous. Content of thought. Delusions. Hallucinations. Illusions. Orientation. Confabulation.

SUMMARY

In one paragraph summarize the essential positive findings in both the history and physical examination, including vital signs.

PROVISIONAL DIAGNOSES

The disease of first importance (primary diagnosis) should be named first. List all major diseases or possibilities in the differential diagnoses. Special examinations and tests (accessory clinical findings) to prove or rule out provisional diagnoses must be ordered by the examining physician. The results of all tests are recorded in a prescribed manner and become a part of the medical record.

Example of manner of writing provisional diagnoses:

1. Undiagnosed lesion of larynx (rule out tbc, chronic infection, neoplasm, lues).

2. Generalized arteriosclerosis.

3. Obesity due to food.

SUGGESTIONS

Treatment: Write a brief statement of the planned approach to treating the problems.

Example: Voice rest and biopsy. Diuresis followed by salt-restricted diet and reduced physical activity.

SPECIAL EXAMINATIONS

Accessory clinical findings: Routine laboratory tests done with each complete physical examination are urinalysis, hemoglobin (Hgb), total white blood cell count (WBC) and differential count of the white blood cells.

Examples of special laboratory reports often necessary are: Blood culture; Sputum or feces examination; Examination of stomach content; Spinal fluid; Special cultures on purulent lesions; Blood urea nitrogen (BUN) and phenolsulfonphthalein (PSP) tests; OT tests for tuberculosis; Liver and bone marrow biopsies; Electrocardiogram (EKG); Electroencephalogram (EEG); Endoscopy (bronchoscopy, cystoscopy); Radiological examinations; Consultations.

FINAL CLINICAL IMPRESSIONS

Final clinical impressions are the diagnoses made after all examinations, special studies and consultations have been noted and considered. They should be written in preferred diagnostic terminology using *Standard Nomenclature of Diseases and Operations* as the proper reference. Here again, the disease of first importance (primary diagnosis) should be named first.

DISPOSITION

As a result of all the foregoing examinations and decisions, a last paragraph should be added stating recommendations which are given the patient. These include drugs and dosages ordered, hospitalization and surgical procedures advised and home care and follow-up visits needed. A remark on the prognosis is also in order.

Chapter IX

ABBREVIATIONS AND SYMBOLS

THERE ARE many constituent parts which combine to make up the finished product of any language. Abbreviations are important and are a special feature of all professional jargons. To understand them signifies a higher degree of knowledge of a profession. They are useful and time-saving in both writing and speaking methods of description.

The medical language is no exception in this respect, and we find many short cuts by utilization of abbreviations. In speaking of temperature, pulse and respiration, for instance, if we abbreviate by T.P.R., we condense ten syllables into three; in writing, we save twenty-seven letters.

The embarrassing phase of the application of abbreviations, however, is the confusing and confounding habit which users make of self-innovated ones. This is done more in writing abbreviations. They are thought up at the moment to suit a special need, but more often produced because the writer is in a hurry to complete his work. It is a hazardous practice since others may ask the interpretation, note it and employ it. This type of abbreviation is of local value only and, if used outside the realm of comprehension, creates difficult tasks of unraveling. They are hazardous, too, because of the fact that a similar abbreviation might have been previously established in a more legitimate use.

It is true that abbreviations, like words, are formed and established because of necessity, and not all result from abused privileges in the forming process. In this chapter are listed both types, but they are those which, from experience, are known to be used in more than a single locale.

Abbreviations and symbols marked "1" in the following pages are legitimately in use or approved. They are to be found in textbooks or dictionaries. Those marked "2" are in general use and might possibly (in the author's opinion) find their way into approved textbooks and dictionaries. Those marked "3" are not approved, and have been coined for local use. Both "2" and "3" may be used only when accompanied by footnotes on interpretation.

The list of abbreviations here is not sufficiently complete to cover all legitimate or coined applications. It is a list of those which the author has found in extensive use.

Abbreviation	Meaning
A.A. (a.a.) [1]	Of each
A.B.C. [1]	Axiobuccocervical
Abdom. [1]	Abdomen
A.B.G. [1]	Axiobuccogingival
A.B.L. [1]	Axiobuccolingual
a.c. [1]	*Ante cibum* = before meals
A.C. [1]	Air conduction
A.C. and B.C. [1]	Air and bone conduction (as in Weber's test)
Acc. [1]	Accommodation
A.C.D. [1]	Absolute cardiac dullness
A.C.E. [1]	Adrenocortical extract
A.C.F. [2]	Accessory clinical findings
A.C.R. [3]	Anticonstipation regime
A.C.S. [1]	American College of Surgeons
ACTH [1]	Adrenocorticotrophic hormone
A.D. [1]	*Auris dextra* = right ear
add. [1]	*Adde* = add; let there be added
ad lib. [1]	*Ad libitum* = at pleasure; at discretion
Adv. [1]	*Adversum* = against

Abbreviation	*Meaning*
Aeg. [1]	*Aegrus* or *aegra* = the patient
aet [1]	At the age of
A.F. [3]	Acid-fast
A/G ratio [1]	Albumin-globulin ratio
$AgNO_3$ [1]	Silver nitrate
ah. [1]	Hypermetropic astigmatism
A.H.A. [1]	American Hospital Association
A.I. [2]	Aortic insufficiency
A.J. [1]	Ankle jerks
Alb. [2]	Albumin
Alt. dieb. [1]	*Alternis diebus* = every other day
Alt. hor. [1]	*Alternis horis* = every other hour
Alt. noct. [1]	*Alternis noctibus* = every other night
A.M. [1]	*Ante meridiem* = before noon
A.M.A. [1]	American Medical Association
amh. [1]	Mixed astigmatism with exceeding myopia
an. [1]	Anisometropia (eyes which require different refractive corrections)
Anes. [1]	Anesthesia
Ante [1]	*Ante* = before
$A_2 > P_2$ [1]	Aortic 2nd heart sound is greater than pulmonic 2nd sound
$A_2 < P_2$ [1]	Aortic 2nd heart sound is less than pulmonic 2nd sound
A.P. [1]	Anterior pituitary
A.P. [3]	Anteroposterior
aq. [1]	*Aqua* = water
aq. com. [1]	*Aqua communis* = common water

Abbreviation	*Meaning*
aq. dist. [1]	*Aqua distillata* = distilled water
As. [1]	Arsenic
a.s. [1]	*Auris sinistra* = left ear
A.S. [2]	Aortic stenosis
As. H. [1]	Hypermetropic astigmatism
As. M. [1]	Myopic astigmatism
A.S.S. [1]	Anterior superior spine
Ast. [1]	Astigmatism
A.T.S. [1]	Antitetanic serum
A.V. [1]	Auriculoventricular
ax. [1]	Axis
A.Z. Test [2]	Aschheim-Zondek test for pregnancy
B. [1]	Bacillus
Ba. [1]	Barium
Bact. [1]	Bacterium
Ba. enem. [1]	Barium enema
B.B.A. [3]	Born before arrival
B.C. [1]	Bone conduction
Benz. [2]	Benzidine
bib. [1]	*Bibe* = drink
b.i.d. [1]	*Bis in die* = twice a day
B.J. [3]	Biceps jerk
B.M. [2]	Bowel movement
B.M.R. [1]	Basal metabolic rate
B.O.A. [3]	Born on arrival
Bol. [1]	*Bolus* = pill

Abbreviation	*Meaning*
B.P. [1]	Blood pressure
B.P.H. [2]	Benign prostatic hypertrophy
B.S. [1]	Breath sounds
B. & S. [3]	Bartholin and Skene glands
B.S.S. [3]	Black silk sutures
B.T. (b.t.) [3]	Brain tumor
BUN [1]	Blood urea nitrogen
$\bar{c}$. [1]	*Cum* = with
C. [1]	Centigrade
C_1; C_2; etc. [1]	First cervical vertebra; Second cervical vertebra; etc.
Ca. [2]	Carcinoma
cal. [1]	Small calorie
Cal. [1]	Large calorie
Cap. [1]	*Capiat* = let him take
cap. [2]	*Capsula* = capsule
Cardio. [2]	Cardiology
Cath. [1]	Cathartic
c.b.c. [1]	Complete blood count
cc. [1]	Cubic centimeters
C.C. [1]	Chief complaint
cd. [1]	Caudal or coccygeal
C.D.C. [3]	Calculated date of confinement
cf. [1]	Compare, or refer to
C.F.T. [1]	Complement-fixation test
CHI_3 [1]	Iodoform
chr. [2]	Chronic

Abbreviation	Meaning
C.I. [1]	Color index
cm. [1]	Centimeter
C.M. [1]	*Cras mane* = tomorrow morning
c.m. [2]	Costal margin
C.N. [1]	*Cras nocte* = tomorrow night
C.N.S. [1]	Central nervous system
CO_2 [1]	Carbon dioxide
Cont. [1]	*Contusus* = bruised
C.P.C. [2]	Clinical Pathological Conference
Cs. [1]	Consciousness
C.S.F. [1]	Cerebrospinal fluid
Cuj. [1]	*Cujus* = of which
C.V. [1]	*Cras vespere* = tomorrow evening
C.V. [2]	Cardiovascular
C.V.A. [2]	Cerebrovascular accident
c.v.a. [2]	Costovertebral angle
C.V.R. [2]	Cardiovascular-respiratory
Cx. [1]	Convex
cyl. [1]	Cylindrical lens
D_1; D_2; etc. [1]	First dorsal vertebra; Second dorsal vertebra; etc.
D.A.H. [1]	Disordered action of heart
D. & C. [2]	Dilation and curettage
D. Cx. [1]	Double convex
D.D. [3]	Dry dressing
decub. [1]	*Decubitus* = lying down
De d. in d. [1]	*De die in diem* = from day to day

Abbreviation	*Meaning*
Deg. [1]	Degree; degeneration
Deglut. [1]	*Deglutiatur* = let it be swallowed
De R [1]	Reaction of degeneration
Derm. [2]	Dermatology
Det. in dup. [1]	*Detur in duplo* = let twice as much be given
Dieb. alt. [1]	*Diebus alternis* = on alternate days
Dieb. tert. [1]	*Diebus tertiis* = every third day
diff. [1]	Differential blood count
dil. [1]	*Dilutus* = dilute; *dilue* = dissolve
Dim. [1]	One-half
div. [1]	Divide
D.M.F. [1]	Decayed, missing and filled teeth
D.O.A. [1]	Dead on arrival
D.P.D. [2]	Department of Public Dispensary
dr. [1]	*Drachma* = dram
D.S.C. [1]	Doctor of Surgical Chiropody
D.T.D. [1]	Dispense of such doses
D.T.N. [1]	Diphtheria toxin normal
Dur. dolor [1]	While the pain lasts
d.v. [1]	Double vibrations
DX (Dx) [2]	Diagnosis
E.A.H.F. [3]	Eczema, allergy, hay fever
ecg [1]	Electrocardiogram
E.C.T. [1]	Electric convulsive treatment
E.D.C. [3]	Expected (or estimated) date of confinement
E.E.G. [1]	Electroencephalogram, -graph

Abbreviation	Meaning
E.E.N.T. [1]	Eye, ear, nose and throat
e.g. [3]	*Exempli gratia* = for example
E.J. [1]	Elbow jerk
EK, EKG, Ekg [1]	Electrocardiogram, -graph
Em. [1]	Emmetropia (normal vision)
Endocrin. [3]	Endocrinology
E.N.T. [1]	Ear, nose and throat
E.O.M. [2]	Extraocular movements
E.S.R. [1]	Erythrocyte sedimentation rate
Etiol [2]	Etiology
ext. [1]	*Extractum* = extract; e.g., *ext. fl.* = fluid extract
F. [1]	Fahrenheit
F.A.C.P. [1]	Fellow, American College of Physicians
F.A.C.S. [1]	Fellow, American College of Surgeons
F. and R. [1]	Force and rhythm (of pulse)
F.B. (f.b.) [2]	Fingerbreadth
F.D. [1]	Focal distance
F.H. [2]	Family history
F.H.S. (f.h.s.) [2]	Fetal heart sounds
Fl. (fld.) [1]	*Fluidum* = fluid
fl. dr. [1]	Fluid dram
F.L.K. [3]	Funny looking kid
Fl. oz. [1]	Fluid ounce
fluor. [3]	Fluoroscopy
F.P. [2]	Flat plate
Fried. Test [3]	Friedman test for pregnancy

Abbreviation	*Meaning*
F.S.H. (FSH) [1]	Follicle-stimulating hormone
ft. [1]	Foot (12 inches)
G.B. [2]	Gallbladder
GC. [2]	Gonorrhea
G.E. [3]	Gastroenterology
Gen'l. [2]	Generalized
G.G.E. [2]	Generalized glandular enlargement
G.I. [1]	Gastrointestinal
gm. [1]	Gram
G.O.E. [2]	Gas, oxygen and ether anesthesia
G.P. [1]	General practitioner
G.P., or G.P.I. [1]	General paresis, or general paralysis of the insane
gr. [1]	*Granum* = grain
G.S.W. [1]	Gunshot wound
gt. [1]	*Gutta* = drop
gtt. [1]	*Guttae* = drops
G.U. [2]	Genitourinary (urogenital)
G.V. [3]	Gentian violet
Gyn. [2]	Gynecology
h. [1]	*Hora* = hour
Hb. [1]	Hemoglobin
HCl [1]	Hydrochloric acid
H.C.V.D. [1]	Hypertensive cardiovascular disease
H.d. [1]	*Hora decubitus* = at bedtime
H.D. [1]	Hearing distance
Hg [1]	*Hydrargyrum* = mercury

Abbreviation	*Meaning*
Hgb. [1]	Hemoglobin
H_2O [1]	Water
H. + Hm. [1]	Compound hypermetropic astigmatism
/HPF [1]	Per high-power field
h.s. [1]	*Hora somni* = at bedtime
H.V.D. [1]	Hypertensive vascular disease
Hx [2]	History
Hy. [1]	Hypermetropia
Id. (id.) [1]	*Idem* = the same
I.M. [1]	Intramuscular
Imp. [2]	Impression
in. [1]	Inch
In d. (in d.) [1]	*In dies* = daily
in extremis [1]	At the point of death
inf. [1]	Infected
inj. [1]	Injection
Int. Med. [1]	Internal Medicine
I.Q. [1]	Intelligence quotient
I.S. [1]	Intercostal space
I.V. [2]	Intravenous
J.J. [3]	Jaw jerk
Kg. [1]	Kilogram (2.2 pounds)
K.I. [1]	Krönig's isthmus
KI [1]	Potassium iodide
k.j. [1]	Knee jerk
k.k. [1]	Knee kick
K.L. bac. [1]	Klebs-Loeffler bacillus (diphtheria)

Abbreviation	Meaning
K.U.B. [1]	Kidney, ureter and bladder
L. (l.) [1]	Liter
L_1; L_2; etc. [1]	First lumbar vertebra; Second lumbar vertebra; etc.
L. & A. (l/a) [1]	Light and accommodation (this is a reaction of the pupils)
Lat. (lat.) [2]	Lateral
lb. [1]	Pound
L.B.D. [2]	Left border of dullness (of heart to percussion)
L.C.M. [2]	Left costal margin
L.H. [1]	Luteinizing hormone
L.I.F. [1]	Left iliac fossa
liq. [1]	*Liquor* = a liquid solution; liquid
L.L. [3]	Large lymphocytes
L.L.Q. [2]	Left lower quadrant
L.M.D. [2]	Local medical doctor
L.M.P. [2]	Last menstrual period
L.O.A. [1]	Left occipitoanterior
L.S.K. [2]	Liver, spleen and kidneys
Lt. (lt.) [1]	Left
L.U.Q. [2]	Left upper quadrant
L. & W. [2]	Living and well
M. [3]	Monocytes
M_1 [2]	Mitral first sound
M.A. [1]	Mental age
M + Am. [1]	Compound myopic astigmatism
Man. pr. [1]	*Mane primo* = eary in the morning

Abbreviation	*Meaning*
McB. pt. [2]	McBurney's point
M.C.H.C. [3]	Mean corpuscular hemoglobin count
M.C.L. [2]	Mid-clavicular line
M.C.V. [2]	Mean corpuscular volume
Med. [1]	Medicine (or medical)
mg. [1]	Milligram
M.H. [2]	Marital history
M.I. [2]	Mitral insufficiency
Mic. [2]	Microscopic findings of centrifuged urinary sediment
min. [1]	*Minim* = one-sixtieth of a dram
M.M. [1]	Mucous membranes
mm. [1]	Millimeter
mm. Hg [1]	Millimeters of mercury
M.S. [2]	Mitral stenosis
M.S.L. [1]	Mid-sternal line
My. [1]	Myopia
NaCl [1]	Sodium chloride (common salt)
N.A.D. [1]	No appreciable disease
N. and V. [2]	Nausea and vomiting
N.B. [2]	Newborn
N.C.A. [1]	Neurocirculatory asthenia
neg. [1]	Negative
Neuro. [2]	Neurology
N_2O [1]	Nitrous oxide
No. (no.) [1]	*Numero* = number
noct. [1]	*Nocte* = at night

Abbreviation	*Meaning*
N.P.N. [1]	Nonprotein nitrogen
N. Surg. [2]	Neurosurgery
N.T.P. [1]	Normal temperature and pressure
Nv. [1]	Naked vision
O.B. (Ob.) (Obs.) [1]	Obstetrics
O.B.-Gyn. [2]	Obstetrics and Gynecology
O.D. [1]	*Oculus dexter* = right eye
ol. [1]	*Oleum* = oil
ol. oliv. [1]	Olive oil
omn. hor. [1]	*Omni hora* = every hour
omn. noct. (o.n.) [1]	*Omni nocte* = every night
O.O.B. [3]	Out of bed
O.P.C. [2]	Outpatient clinic
O.P.D. [2]	Outpatient dispensary
Ophth. [2]	Ophthalmology
O.R. [2]	Operating room
Orth. [2]	Orthopedics
O.S. (o.s.) [1]	*Oculus sinister* = left eye
Osteo. [3]	Osteomyelitis
O.T. [1]	Old tuberculin
Oto. [3]	Otology
O.U. [1]	*Oculus uterque* = each eye
Ov. [1]	*Ovum* = egg
oz. [1]	Ounce
P. [1]	Pulse
P_2 [1]	Pulmonic second sound
P. & A. [2]	Percussion and auscultation

Abbreviation	Meaning
P. æ. [1]	*Partes aequales* = in equal parts
P-a-ra [1]	Pregnancies (e.g., Para 4-1-2 = 4 pregnancies, 1 abortion or miscarriage, 2 living children)
Para I [1]	A woman having borne one child (unipara)
Para II [1]	A woman having borne two children (bipara)
Par. aff. [1]	*Pars affecta* = the part affected
PAT [2]	Paroxysmal auricular tachycardia
Path. [2]	Pathology
P.C. (p.c.) [1]	*Post cibum* = after meals
PcB [1]	Near point of convergence
p.d. [1]	Interpapillary distance or papilla diameter
P.D. [1]	Potential difference
P.D.C. [2]	Private diagnostic clinic
P.E. [2]	Physical examination
Ped. [2]	Pediatrics
P.H. [2]	Past history
Phys. Med. [2]	Physical Medicine
P.I. [2]	Present illness
P.I.D. [2]	Pelvic inflammatory disease
P.L. (p.l.) [1]	Light perception
P.M. [3]	*Post mortem* = after death
P.M. (p.m.) [1]	*Post meridiem* = after noon
P.M.B. [1]	Polymorphonuclear basophilic leukocytes
P.M.E. [1]	Polymorphonuclear eosinophilic leukocytes
P.M.I. [1]	Point of maximal impulse (of heart on chest wall)

Abbreviation	Meaning
P.M.N. [1]	Polymorphonuclear neutrophilic leukocytes
P.M.P. [2]	Previous menstrual period
P.N. [1]	Percussion note
P.N.D. [2]	Postnasal drip
Polio. [1]	Poliomyelitis, epidemic
P. Op. [2]	Postoperative
PPD. [1]	Purified protein derivative of tuberculin
p.r.n. [1]	*Pro re nata* = whenever necessary
Prog. [2]	Prognosis
P.S.P. [1]	Phenolsulfonphthalein test (kidney)
P. Surg. [2]	Plastic Surgery
Psy. [3]	Psychiatry
Psych. [3]	Psychology
pt. [3]	Patient
P.T. [3]	Physical therapy
pulv. [1]	Powder
P.U.O. [1]	Pyrexia of undetermined origin
Px. [1]	Pneumothorax
P.X. (Px) [3]	Physical examination
P.Z.I. [3]	Protamine zinc insulinate
q.d. [3]	*Quaque die* = every day
q.h. [1]	*Quaque hora* = every hour
q.i.d. [1]	*Quater in die* = four times a day
q.n. [3]	*Quaque nocte* = every night
q.q. hor. [1]	*Quaque hora* = every hour
q.s. [1]	*Quantum sufficit* = enough; a sufficient quantity

Abbreviation	*Meaning*
q.v. [1]	*Quantum vis* = as much as you like
R. [1]	Respiration
R. (r.) (Rt.) [1]	Right
Ra [1]	Radium
R.B.C. [1]	Red blood cells (red blood count)
R.B.D. [2]	Right border of dullness (of heart to percussion)
R.C.D. [1]	Relative cardiac dullness
R.C.M. [2]	Right costal margin
R.D. [1]	Reaction of degeneration
R.E.S. [1]	Reticuloendothelial system
R.H.D. [1]	Relative hepatic dullness
Rh. neg. [1]	Rhesus factor negative
R.I.F. [1]	Right iliac fossa
R.L.Q. [2]	Right lower quadrant
R.L.S. person. [1]	Person who stammers, being unable to enunciate R, L, and S
R.M. [1]	Respiratory movement
R.M.D. [3]	Retromanubrial dullness
Rn [1]	Radon
R.O.A. [1]	Right occipitoanterior
Rom. [3]	Romberg
R.O.P. [1]	Right occipitoposterior
R.O.S. [2]	Review of systems
R. R. & E. [2]	Round, regular and equal (of pupils)
R. units [1]	Roentgen units
R.U.Q. [2]	Right upper quadrant

Abbreviation	Meaning
R.V. [3]	Retroversion
R.V.O. [3]	Relaxed vaginal outlet
$\overline{\text{s}}$. [1]	*Sine* = without
S. [1]	Sacral vertebrae
sig. [1]	*Signetur* = let it be labeled
S.L. [3]	Small lymphocytes
S.M.D. [3]	Submanubrial dullness
S.M.W.D.Sep. [2]	Single, married, widowed, divorced, separated
S.O.B. [2]	Shortness of breath
Sol. [1]	*Solutio* = solution
solv. [1]	Dissolve
S. op. S. (s.o.s.) [1]	*Si opus sit* = if necessary
Sp. gr. [1]	Specific gravity
sph. [1]	Spherical or spherical lens
sq. cell ca. [1]	Squamous cell carcinoma
S.R. [1]	Sedimentation rate (C.S.R.[2] = corrected sedimentation rate.)
s.s. [1]	Soapsuds
SS (ss) [1]	*Semis* = one-half
S.S.V. [1]	*Sub signo veneni* = under a poison label
Staph. [1]	Staphylococcus, -al
Stat. [1]	*Statim* = at once
Stb. [2]	Stillborn
STD [1]	Skin test dose
Stereo. [2]	Stereogram
Stet [1]	Let it stand

Abbreviation	*Meaning*
Str. [1]	Streptococcus, -al
Strab. [3]	Strabismus
STS [1]	Serology tests for syphilis
Subcu. [3]	Subcutaneous
Sug. [2]	Sugar
Surg. [2]	Surgery, surgical, surgeon
Syph. [3]	Syphilology
Syr. [1]	*Syrupus* = syrup
T. [1]	Temperature
T & A [1]	Tonsils and adenoids; tonsillitis and adenoiditis; tonsillectomy and adenoidectomy
T.A.B. [1]	Typhoid, paratyphoid A and paratyphoid B vaccine
T.A.T. [1]	Tetanus antitoxin
Tbc (tbc) [1]	Tuberculosis; tubercle bacilli
temp. dext. [1]	*Tempus dextra* = right temple
T.F. [3]	Tactile fremitus
T.I.D. (t.i.d.) [1]	*Ter in die* = three times a day
tinct. [1]	Tincture
T.J. [1]	Triceps jerk
T.P.R. [2]	Temperature, pulse, respiration
Tr. (tr.) [1]	*Tinctura* = tincture
T.S. [1]	Test solution
Tus. (tus.) [1]	*Tussis* = cough
U.C.H.D. [2]	Usual childhood diseases
U.D. [3]	Urethral discharge
ult. [3]	*Ultimum* = lastly

Abbreviation	*Meaning*
Umb. [1]	*Umbilicus* = navel
Ung. (ung.) [1]	Ointment
Ur. (ur.) [1]	Urine
U.R.I. [2]	Upper respiratory infection
Urol. [2]	Urology
U.S.P. [1]	United States Pharmacopoeia
U.S.P.H.S. [1]	United States Public Health Service
Va. [1]	Visual acuity
Vand. [3]	Van den Bergh (Liver function test)
V. and T. [1]	Volume and tension of pulse
var. [1]	Variety
V.C. [1]	Color vision
V.D. [1]	Venereal disease
V.D.G. [1]	Venereal disease — gonorrhea
V.D.H. [1]	Valvular disease of heart
V.D.S. [1]	Venereal disease — syphilis
Ves. ur. [1]	*Vesica urinaria* = urinary bladder
V.f. [1]	Vision field (field of vision)
V.F. [1]	Vocal fremitus
viz. [1]	*Videlicet* = namely
V.R. [1]	Vocal resonance
V.W. [1]	Vessel wall
W.B.C. (w.b.c.) [1]	White blood cells (white blood count)
w-d [2]	Well-developed
W.F. [2]	White female
W.M. [2]	White male
w-n [3]	Well-nourished

Abbreviation	Meaning
Wt. [1]	Weight
X. [1]	Unit of X-ray dosage
y.s. [1]	A yellow spot (on retina)

SYMBOLS

m	*misce* = mix
ℳ	minim
°	degree
O̅	pint
ℨ	dram
℥	ounce
*	birth
†	death
—	negative
+	positive
±	positive or negative
♂ or □	male
♀ or ○	female
c̄	together with
s̄	without

REFERENCE

Morris Fishbein, *Medical Writing* (2nd ed.; Philadelphia: The Blakiston Co., 1948).

CHAPTER X

MEDICAL EQUIVALENTS OF LAY TERMINOLOGY

Lay Terminology	Medical Terminology
Adam's apple	prominentia laryngea
afterbirth	placenta and membranes; secundines
ague	chill; usually with malarial fever
ain't seen nothing	amenorrhea; menstruation has ceased
air or altitude sickness	anoxia
air swallowing	aerophagia
appearance, old in	progeria
appearance, young in	agerasia
appetite, loss of	anorexia
armpit	axilla
athlete's foot	dermatophytosis
baby, unborn	fetus
bad blood	syphilis; lues
bag of waters	amniotic sac; amnion
baldness	alopecia
baldness in patches	alopecia areata
ball-and-socket joint	enarthrosis
barber's itch	tinea barbae; sycosis vulgaris; sycosis barbae
baseball finger	fracture—sprain of distal phalanx
bealing in ear	otitis media

Note: For additional lay words, see Index.

Lay Terminology	Medical Terminology
bedbug	cimex
bedsore	decubitus ulcer
bed-wetting	enuresis
belching, or burping	eructation; regurgitation
bends or decompression sickness	anoxemia
birth canal	vagina
birthin', or burfin'	act of delivery of child
black eye	ecchymosis about eyelid
blackhead	comedo
blindness, mind	apraxia
night	nyctalopia
partial	meropia
blister or bleb	bulla; cutaneous vesicle
blood blister	subepithelial hematoma
blood poisoning	septicemia
bloody flux	diarrhea, or dysentery with blood content
blue mole	nevus pigmentosus
blue, turning	cyanotic, cyanosis
body	uterus
body trouble	any gynecological disease
boil	furuncle (or furunculosis)
bone felon	osteomyelitis of tip of finger
born with teeth	dentia praecox
bowel movement, bloody or bloody stools	hematochezia
bowleg	genu varum

Lay Terminology	*Medical Terminology*
boxer's fracture	fracture of fifth metacarpal
boxer's fracture 5th finger	fracture distal head 5th metacarpal
brain fever	meningitis; encephalitis
breath, bad	fetor oris
Bright's disease	glomerular nephritis
bruise	contusion
bunion	hallux valgus
buttox, fat	steatopygia
canker sores	ulcerations of mouth
carbolic acid	phenol
carbuncle	subcutaneous abscess around hair follicles (usually on back or posterior neck)
cat fever	upper respiratory infection, acute
cauliflower ear or broken cartilage of ear with effusion	chondrodystrophy of ear, traumatic
change of life	climacteric; menopause
charleyhorse	contusion or overstrain of muscle
charms	labia minora
chewing	masticating
childbed fever	puerperal septicemia
chills; usually malaria	ague
chin, receding or small; Andy Gump chin	micrognathia
cholera morbus	diarrhea
clap	gonorrhea; neisserosis
cold in the head	coryza

Lay Terminology	Medical Terminology
cold, June	usually hay fever
cold sore	herpes simplex
color blindness	achromatopsia; daltonism (inability to distinguish between red and green)
colorless	achromia
connections	intercourse; coition
consumption	tuberculosis
corn	clavus
cradle cap or milk crust	dermatitis seborrheica (usually)
cramp	muscular contraction or spasm
in calf muscle of leg	systremma
creeping paralysis	any slowly progressing paralysis; i.e., progressive muscular dystrophy; multiple sclerosis
crick in neck	acute torticollis
cross-eyes	strabismus
croup	laryngitis
crud (slang for repulsive condition)	exuding pus; common cold
crying	lacrimating
curvature of spine	scoliosis
cut	laceration
dandruff	dermatitis seborrheica
dead bone	sequestrum
dimple, chin	symphysis menti
discomfort or distress, vague	general malaise

Lay Terminology	*Medical Terminology*
disease, aftereffects	sequelae
approach or beginning of	prodromal stage
distention of stomach or intestines due to air or gases	flatulence
drawing spell	convulsion; epilepsy; hyperventilation
dreens	leucorrhea
driver's elbow	bursitis of olecranon
droopy lids	blepharoptosis
dropped womb	descensus uteri; prolapse of uterus
dropsy (abnormal accumulation of fluid in body tissue or cavities)	anasarca (if general) ; or hydrops ascites (if abdominal) edema (may be used in general or specified areas)
dying condition	moribund condition
dyspepsia	gastric disorder or impairment
ear stopped up after flight	aerotitis
earache	otalgia
earwax	cerumen
eating dirt or earth	geophagia
eating rapidly	tachyphagia
eating starch (as in pregnancy)	pica
expecting	pregnant
eyebrow	supercilium
eyestrain or fatigue	asthenopia; ophthalmocopia
false teeth	dentures

Lay Terminology	*Medical Terminology*
farsightedness	hypermetropia
fat	adipose tissue; obese
fear of; dread of; morbid dislike of; aversion or intolerance to	phobia

TYPES OF PHOBIAS:

age, old	gerontophobia
air or drafts	aerophobia
airplanes; *see* heights	
alone, being	monophobia
animals	zoophobia
baldness	peladophobia
beating, a	rhabdophobia
bees	apiphobia
blood, sight of	hemaphobia
bridge, walking on; or near water	gephyrophobia
cancer	cancerophobia
cats	ailurophobia; galeophobia; gatophobia
childbirth	tocophobia
children	pedophobia
closed-in spaces or confined	claustrophobia
colors	chromatophobia
crowds	koinoniphobia
darkness or night	noctiphobia; nyctophobia; scotophobia
death	thanatophobia

Lay Terminology	*Medical Terminology*
doctors	iatrophobia
dogs	kynophobia (rabies = hydrophobia)
drafts; *see* air	
dust	coniophobia
eat	sitophobia
fat, being	lipophobia
fatigue; *see* work	
fever	febriphobia
filth	rhypophobia; rupophobia
fire	pyrophobia
God, wrath of	theophobia
heat or tropics	thermophobia
heights	acrophobia; hypsophobia
hell	hadephobia
illness	nosophobia
insane persons; *see* lunatics	
insects, stinging	melissophobia
kidnapped, being; *see* thief	
lice	pediculophobia
lightning	keraunophobia
lunatics	demonophobia
male sex; *see* sex	
microbes	microphobia
moisture	hygrophobia
new things	neophobia

Lay Terminology	*Medical Terminology*
fear of — *Continued*	
night; *see* darkness	
number 13	triskaidekaphobia
odors	olfactophobia
old age; *see* age	
open spaces	agoraphobia
pain	algophobia
parasites	parasitophobia
phobias, one's own	phobophobia
phone, talking on	telephonophobia
poisons	toxicophobia
poverty	peniaphobia
responsibility, assuming	hypengyophobia
rivers, crossing or streams; *see also* bridges	potamophobia
sex, male	androphobia
sexual love	erotophobia
snakes	ophidiophobia
speaking (especially if one stutters)	lalophobia
strangers	xenophobia
syphilis	syphilophobia
talking in public; *see* speaking	
temperature rise; *see* fever	
thief, of becoming a, or of being kidnapped	kleptophobia

Lay Terminology	*Medical Terminology*
things, multiple	polyphobia
thirteen; *see* number 13	
touched, being	haphephobia
trains, riding in	siderodromophobia
tuberculosis	phthisiophobia
venereal infection	venereophobia
women, society of	gynephobia
work or being fatigued	ponophobia
feeling life	first fetal movement
felon; *see* whitlow	
fever	febrile condition; pyrexia
childbirth	puerperal endometritis or metritis
red	erysipelas
snail	schistosomiasis
swamp or marsh	malaria
sweat	miliaria
fever blister	herpes simplex
fingerprints	dactylographs or grams
fits	convulsion
flat foot	pes valgoplanus
flea bites	pulicosis (flea = pulex) ; pulex irritans
floating kidney	nephroptosis
flooding	menorrhagia
flux	diarrhea; dysentery
foreskin	prepuce

Lay Terminology	Medical Terminology
fragrant	pregnant
freckle	ephelis (pl. = ephelides)
funny bone	the sensitive spot in the elbow joint where ulnar nerve runs superficially between olecranon and coronoid processes
funnygrams, medical	errors in interpretation of (usually dictated) medical terms. (e.g., tending sheep for *tendon sheath;* funnel headed for *frontal headache;* B - 9 tumor for *benign tumor*)
galloping consumption	miliary tuberculosis
gas or air in stomach and intestines	flatus
glimmer	scotomata; dimness of visual acuity
goose flesh	cutis anserina
granulated eyelids	trachoma
gravel in gallbladder	cholecystolithiasis
gravel in kidney	nephrolithiasis
groin	inguinal region
growing pains (in children)	rheumatism (usually)
gumboil	epulis; parulis
hair, dry	xerasia
falling	lipsotrichia
graying	poliothrix
rapid loss of	trichorrhea
haircut	penile chancre
hairy	hirsute
hammertoe	flexion deformity of toe joint

Lay Terminology	Medical Terminology
hamstring	the biceps tendinosus and semimembranous tendons
hangnail, infected	paronychia
hawking and snorting	screatus
hay fever	allergic rhinitis
headache, sick	migraine
heart attack	usually implies coronary artery occlusion
heartburn	pyrosis
heatstroke or sunstroke	siriasis; thermoplegia
hexed (to be accursed, to be cast under the spell of one who is seeking vengeance; hypnotism in a sense)	a type of psychosis
hiccup	singultus
high blood	hypertension
hind baby	breech delivery
hip baby (hip-tall to mother)	second to youngest walking sibling (usually 3rd child)
hives	urticaria
honeymoon appendicitis	acute cystitis or urethritis seen in young brides
hookworm	ancylostomiasis
housemaid's knee	bursitis of knee
hunchback, or humpback	kyphosis
hunger, abnormal	limosis
hydrophobia	rabies
ill in bed	bedridden

Lay Terminology	*Medical Terminology*
in the family way	pregnant
infanticipating (Winchell)	pregnant
infantile paralysis	anterior poliomyelitis
ingrown toenail	unguis incarnatus
iron deficiency	sideropenia
itch	pruritus
mad	urticaria
jaw, protruding	macrognathia
joint mouse	loose body in joint
jungle rot	fungus infection
knee baby (knee-high to mother)	next youngest sibling
knock-kneed	genu valgum
labor (or delivery of child), difficult or slow	dystocia
lead poisoning	plumbism
leaking heart	heart murmur; valvular disease
leg ache	intermittent claudication; causalgia
lice	pediculosis (of body: p. corporis; of head: p. capitis; of pubis: p. pubis)
lightening	descent of uterus into pelvic cavity two to three weeks before labor begins; engagement of fetal head
liver fluke	opisthorchis viverrini
liver spots	chloasms
locked bowels	intestinal obstruction (i.e., paralytic ileus, etc.)

Lay Terminology	*Medical Terminology*
lockjaw	tetanus
long life or longevity	macrobiosis
low blood	anemia; or hypotension
lumbago	painful back; might be myositis, over-strain of joint, etc.
lump in the throat	globus hystericus
lying face downward	prone position
lying face up (on back)	supine position; supination
mad itch	urticaria
mange	probably psoriasis or dermatitis seborrheica
matter	pus
measles, baby German, or three-day red	roseola rubella rubeola
mental state of great calm — freedom from anxiety	psychodelic
midriff	region of diaphragm
milk leg	phlegmasia alba dolens
milk rash	eczema
mindreader	telepathist
miner's elbow	bursitis of olecranon
miscarriage	abortion (usually early)
misery	pain
mishap	abortion
mite	acarus (pl. = acari) ; acariasis

Lay Terminology	*Medical Terminology*
moles	nevi (the type must be described; i.e., nevus pigmentosus; nevus pilosus)
morning sickness	hyperemesis gravidarum
movement, loss of or paralysis	akinesia
mumps	epidemic parotitis
nail biting	onychophagia
nails, breaking	onychoclasis
white discoloration	leukonychia
narrowing or stricture	stenosis
nearsightedness	myopia
night blindness	nyctalopia
nightmare or night terrors	pavor nocturnus
nose stopped up	hypertrophic rhinitis
nosebleed	epistaxis
numbness	paresthesia
openings	introitus; meatus; mouth; orifice; os; vestibule
out of head	delirium
outline	schema
ovals	ovaries
pain, referred	telalgia
parrot fever	psittacosis
patches, brown moth of skin	chloasma
white of skin or piebald skin	leukoderma; vitiligo

Lay Terminology	*Medical Terminology*
perspiration, profuse	hyperhidrosis; sudoresis; sudorrhea
phlegm	mucus
phobias	*see* fears
pigeon toe	forefoot varus
piles	hemorrhoids
pink eye	conjunctivitis, infectious
pip jinnie	furuncle
pipping	metrorrhagia
playboy (or sport) or freak of nature	lusus naturae
pointed head	oxycephaly
poker back or poker spine	spondylitis deformans
policeman's heel	bursitis of heel or painful heel
porter's bursa	subacromial bursitis
prickly heat	miliaria
puke	emesis
punch drunk	cerebral concussion usually
pupils, dilation of	mydriasis
inequality in diameter	anisocoria
inequality of vision	anisopis
small	microcoria
quickening	feeling fetal life
quilling (in home deliveries) by use of a goose quill during delivery	producing sternutation (sneezing)
quinsy	peritonsillar abscess

Lay Terminology	*Medical Terminology*
rabbit fever	tularemia
railroad spine	post-traumatic painful back, sometimes called vertebral injury (compensationitis)
rat bite fever	sokosha
reading difficulty	dyslexia
ringing in ears	tinnitus
ringworm	tinea (specify type)
rising, a	abscess
rising in ear	otitis media
run-around	paronychia
saber shins	anterior bowing tibia (usually syphilitic) with hypertrophy anterior cortex; may be result of rickets with hypertrophy posterior cortex
saddleback	lordosis
St. Vitus' dance	chorea
saliva, excessive secretion of	ptyalism
scalded butt	excoriated buttocks
seasickness	mal de mer; naupathia
seen nothing	amenorrhea
sense of well-being or body comfort	euphoria (used in psychiatry as an exaggerated sense)
shinbone	tibia
shingles	herpes zoster
shootin' in	beginning of lactation in new mother (about 3rd day following delivery)

Lay Terminology	*Medical Terminology*
sif	syphilis; lues
skin, dry	xeroderma
peeling or shedding	desquamation
yellowish discoloration	xanthosis
sleeping sickness	encephalitis lethargica
sleepwalking	somnambulism
smallpox	variola
snail fever; *see* fever	
snapping hip	slipping tensor fascia lata over trochanter
snapping jaw	dislocation of meniscus of jaw
snapping jaws	deranged intra-articular cartilage temporomandibular joint
snoring	stertor; stertorous or sonorous breathing
social diseases	gonorrhea or syphilis (lues)
softening	malacia
solid	stereo- (prefix)
sour stomach	impairment of digestion
spasm of eyelid	tic or habit spasm
speech impairment	dyslalia
spit	expectoration
spitting blood	hemoptysis
spitting up	regurgitation
splayfoot	flatfoot; talipes valgus
spots before eyes	scotomata
spotting	metrorrhagia

Lay Terminology	*Medical Terminology*
stone bruise	plantar contusions (from walking barefoot over rocky ground)
stones in gallbladder	cholecystolithiasis
stones in kidney	nephrolithiasis
store teeth	dentures
strawberry	abrasion of skin
stricture; *see* narrowing	
string-haltered	contracture of achilles tendon
stroke	hemiplegia; rupture of cerebral vessel
stye	hordeolum
sunburn	actinic dermatitis
sunstroke; *see* heatstroke	
swage down	decrease in edema
swayback; *see* saddleback	
sweat	hidrosis
sweat bath	sudarium
sweat or perspiration	sudor
sweating profusely; *see* perspiration	
sweet or sugar diabetes	diabetes mellitus
swelling	edema (usually)
swoon	syncope
tail	cauda
talking, excessive	lalorrhea; logorrhea
teeth, buck	protrusion of upper incisors
grinding	bruxism; stridor dentium
widely separated	hag or rake

Lay Terminology	*Medical Terminology*
tennis elbow	radio-humeral elbow
tetter	dermatitis
the change	climacteric; menopause
thin-skinned	leptodermic
thrash	moniliasis; thrush
tick fever	Rocky Mountain spotted fever
tongue-tie	ankyloglossia
tooth decay	caries of teeth; saprodontia
trick knee	torn meniscus or loose body
trigger finger	hypertrophy flexor tendons with blocking in sheath
twinge	short, sharp pain
up-chuck	emesis
upside-down stomach	thoracic stomach
voice, nasal	rhinophonia
weak	leptophonia
vomit	emesis
wakefulness, abnormal	egersis
wart	verruca
wasting palsy	progressive muscular atrophy
water ball	cyst
water cure	hydrotherapy
water head	hydrocephalus
water on knee	hydrarthrosis
wax in ears	cerumen
weaver's bottom	bursitis of gluteal (ischial) bursa
web-fingers	syndactylism

Lay Terminology	*Medical Terminology*
wen	sebaceous cyst
wheal (a raise or elevation on skin such as might be made by a nail stroke)	dermographia
wheezes	asthma
white cells eating up red cells	leukemia
white leg; *see* milk leg	
white swelling	tuberculous abscess
whitehead	steatoma
whites	leucorrhea
whitlow or felon	paronychia
whooping cough	epidemic pertussis
wink, to	palpebrate
witch's milk	(milk-like secretion from breast of newborn) mastitis neonatorum
worms	vermis (type must be described; i.e., ascariasis, etc.)
wrinkle	rhytis; rhytidosis
excision of	rhytidectomy
writer's cramp	cheirospasm
yellow janders	jaundice (malfunctioning liver, disease to be named)

REFERENCES

An Introduction to Medical Terminology
    by George L. Banay
    Reprints from *Bulletin of Medical Library Association* furnished by
    Dr. Banay

Black's Law Dictionary (3rd edition)
    by Henry K. Black
    West Publishing Company, St. Paul, Minn.

Contribution of Greek to English
    by Charles Barrett Brown
    Vanderbilt University Press, Nashville, Tenn.

Gould's Medical Dictionary (5th revised edition)
    by G. M. Gould
    The Blakiston Company, Philadelphia, Pa.

Madame Claire
    by Susan Ertz
    Appleton-Century-Crofts, Inc., New York City

Medical Etymology
    by O. H. Perry Pepper
    W. B. Saunders Company, Philadelphia, Pa.

Medical Greek (1908 edition)
    by Achilles Rose
    Peri Hellados Publications Office, New York City

Medical Greek and Latin at a Glance (2nd edition)
    by Walter R. Agard
    Paul B. Hoeber, Inc., New York City

Medical Records in the Hospital
    by Malcolm T. MacEachern
    Physicians' Record Company, Berwyn, Ill.

Medical Writing
    by Morris Fishbein
    The Blakiston Company, Philadelphia, Pa.

Origin of Medical Terms
    by Henry Alan Skinner
    Williams and Wilkins Company, Baltimore, Md.

The American Illustrated Medical Dictionary
    by W. A. Newman Dorland
    W. B. Saunders Company, Philadelphia, Pa.

The Directory of Medical Specialists (Vol. 4)
    by Advisory Board for Medical Specialties
    A. N. Marquis Company, Chicago, Ill.

The Language of Medicine
    by R. F. Campbell
    D. Appleton Company, New York City

The Standard Nomenclature of Diseases and Operations (1961 edition)
    Sponsored by The American Medical Association, Chicago, Ill.
    McGraw-Hill Book Company, Inc., New York City

Walter Winchell (Syndicated Column)
    by Walter Winchell
    New York City

Webster's New International Dictionary (2nd edition)
    G. and C. Merriam Company, Springfield, Mass.

INDEX

INDEX

A

A-, 31; 135; 136; 137; 140; 141; 142

$\overline{\text{A.A.}}$ (a.a.), 210

Ab-, 28; 116; 135

Abasia, 135

Abbreviations and symbols, 209

A.B.C., 210

Abdom., 210

Abdomen, 10; 205; 210

Abdominal: see ventral, 190

Abdominal and pelvic wall lining = parietal peritoneum, 78; 79

Abdominal cavity, fluid in: see ascites, 141

Abdominal cavity lining = peritoneum, 63

Abdominal pain: see under gastrointestinal, 198

Abdominal regions and operational incisions, 59

Abduct, 135

Abductor pollicis brevis, 88

Aberrant, 135

A.B.G., 210

Ability: see -able; -ible, 43

A.B.L., 210

Ablation, 51

Ablatio placentae, 116

-able, 43

Abnormal, 28

Abnormality: see anomaly, 140

Abortion, 116; 241

Above: see super-; supra-, 31; sublimis, 89

Abrasion, 135

Abrasion of skin, 246

Abscess, 244

Abscess, peritonsillar, 108; also see quinsy, 243

Abscess, pyoptysis due to, 180

Abscess, retroperitoneal, 63

Abscess, subcutaneous around hair follicles, 231

Absent at birth: see agenesis, 136

Absolute cardiac dullness, 210

-ac, 43

A.C. (a.c.), 210

A.C. and B.C., 210

Acariasis, 135

Acariasis of scalp, 135

Acarus, 241

Acc., 210

Accessory clinical findings: see A.C.F., 207; 210

Accommodation, 210

A.C.D., 210

A.C.E., 210

Acetabulum, 84

Acetone, 135

A.C.F., 210

Achalasia, 135

Achalasia of sphincter of esophagus: see achalasia, 135

Achilles tendon, contracture of: see string-haltered, 246

Achne, 80

Acholuria, 136

Achondroplasia, 48; 65; 92

Achromatopsia, 129; 232

Achromia, 232

Acid-fast, 211

Acinar tissue, 102

Acinum, 102

Acne, 80

Acoustic sense, 127

A.C.R., 210

Acro-, 36

Acromegaly, 120

Acromion process, 36

Acrophobia, 235

Across: see ana, 28; 138

A.C.S., 210

ACTH, 210

Appetite: see -orexia, 47; 69; orexis, 140; see also under gastro-intestinal, 198

Appetite, loss of = anorexia, 47; 69; 140; 229

Appetite, ravenous: see lycorexia, 168

Appleton-Century-Crofts, Inc., 10; 249

Appleton, D., Company, 250

Application, plaster cast, 58

Apraxia, 141; 230

aq., 211

aq. com., 211

aq. dist., 212

Aqua, 127; 211

Aqua communis, 211

Aqua distillata, 212

Aqueous, 127

Arachne, 122

Arachnoid, 122

Arch: see under mouth and throat, 202

Archlike: see fornix, 159

Arch, zygomatic, 88

Area: see areola, 80

Areas on body, depressed: see fossa, 159

Areolar tissue, subcutaneous, 80

Arising: see oriens, 174

Arm: see brachium, 6

Arm bone, upper = humerus, 85

Armpit = axilla, 229; also see under superficial fossae, 79

Around: see circum-, 29; peri-, 29; 105; 177

Arrow: see sagitta, 125

Arteria, 4; 67

Arteries, hardening of = arteriosclerosis, 67

Arteries of heart, narrowing of = stenocardia, 40

Arteriorrhaphy, 56

Arteriosclerosis, 67; 97

Artery, 4; 67; 97

Artery, coronary, 99

Artery of foot and leg = peroneal, 66

Artery, peroneal, 66

Artery, pulmonary, 99

Artery suspending the heart: see aorta, 140

Artery, suturing of = arteriorrhaphy, 56

Artery walls, thickening of; (hard-ening of) = arteriosclerosis, 67

Arthritis, gonococcal, 93

Arthritis, hypertrophic, 93

Arthritis, rheumatoid, 94

Arthritis, syphilitic, 94

Arthritis, tuberculous, 95

Arthrodesis, 55

Arthron, 64

Artificial leg, eye or part: see pros-thesis, 179

Artificial substitute: see prosthesis, 179

a.s., 212

As., 212

A.S., 212

Ascariasis: see under worms, 248

Aschheim-Zondek test for pregnancy, 212

Ascites, 141; 233; also see under abdomen, 205

Asepsis, 141

As.H., 212

Askos, 141

As.M., 141

As much as you like: see q.v., 224

Aspiration, 50

A.S.S., 212

Ast., 212

Asthenia, 141

Asthenopia, 233

Asthma, 96; see also under allergic tendencies, 197

Astigmatism: see Ast., 212

Astigmatism, compound hyperme-tropic: see under H+Hm., 218

Astigmatism, compound, myopic, 219

Astigmatism, hypermetropic: see ah, 211; also see As. H., 212

Astigmatism, myopic: see As. M., 212

Astragalus: see under tarsal bones, 88

At bedtime, 218

At discretion: see ad lib., 210

Atelectasis, 37; 46; 96

B

Bad blood, 229
Bad breath: see fetor oris, 231
Ba. enem., 212
Baglike: see cyst, 46; 81; 82; 128; sac, 131; 141; 151
Bag of waters, 229
Balance, equal = equilibrium, 33
Balanitis, 112
Balanos, 112
Baldness: see alopecia, 137; 229
Baldness in patches: see alopecia areata, 137; 229
Ball-and-socket joint, 229
Ballottement, 145
Banay, George L., 249
Bandage: see splenion, 91
Barber's itch, 229
Barium, 212
Barium enema, 212
Barrel chest: see under thorax, 203
Bartholin and Skene glands, 213
Basal metabolic rate: see B.M.R., 212
Baseball finger, 229
Base or bottom: see fundus, 160
Basis, 135
Bath, sweat: see sweat bath, 246
B.B.A., 212
B.C., 212
Bealing in ear, 229
Bearing (offspring): see -parous, 33; 47; parere, 117; 171; 179
Bear, to: see parere, 117; gestare, 160
Bed: see kline, 13; 150
Bedbug: see cimex, 230
Bedsore = decubitus ulcer, 81; 152; 230
Bedtime, at: see hora decubitus and hora somni, 217; 218
Bed-wetting: see enuresis, 156; 230
Before: see pre-, 28; 178; 179; ante-, 28; 211; pro-, 28; 179
Before meals: see A.C. (a.c.), 210
Before noon, 211
Behind: see opisthen, 174; postero-, 36
Behind, at the side = postero-lateral, 36

Belching: see eructation, 157; re-gurgitation, 181; 230
Bell's palsy, 92
Belly: see gaster, 89; venter, 190
Bending backward: see retroflexion, 31; opistho-, 36
Bends: see anoxemia, 230
Benign prostatic hypertrophy, 112; 213
Bent: see -vara, 92; kyphos, 165; lordos, 167
Bent forward: see lordosis, 167
Bent or crooked: see ankylos, 139
Bent structure: see genu, 160
Benz., 212
Benzidine, 212
Beside: see para-, 31; 82; 105; 109; 115; 177
Between: see inter-, 30
Bi-, 32; 89; 145
bib., 212
Bibe, 212
Biceps: see under neurological survey, 206
Biceps brachii, 89
Biceps jerk, 212
b.i.d., 212
Bifidus, 94
Bifurcation, 145
Bilateral, 32
Bile: see chole, 68; 103; 105; 136
Bile ducts, inflammation of = cholangitis, 107
Bile ducts, suturing of = choledochorrhaphy, 57
Bile passages, stones in = choleli-thiasis, 44; biliary calculi, 107
Bile pigments in blood = verdohemin, 35
Biliary calculi, 107
Bin-, 32
Bind (make tight): see -desis, 54
Bind, to: see ligare, 90; sphingein, 91; nectere, 136
Binocular, 32
Biochemics, 63
Biochemist, 18
Biochemistry, 18
Biopsies of bone marrow: see under special examinations, 208

Biopsy, 51
Biopsy of lymph node, 51
Bios, 51; 63; 76
Bipara: see Para, 222
Birth: see genesis, 151; natus, 179
birth: see symbol *, 228
Birth, before: see prenatal, 28; 179
Birth canal, 230
Birth, giving: see parturition, 177
Birthin', 230
Birth, with: see congenital, 29; 151
Bis in die, 212
B.J., 212
Black: see melan-, 35
Black eye: see ecchymosis about
    eyelid, 230
Blackhead = comedo, 230
Black, Henry K., 1; 249
Black silk sutures, 213
Black's Law Dictionary, 1; 249
Bladder: see vesica, 110; vesicula,
    111; askos, 141
Bladder, exstrophy of, 112
Bladder, small: see vesicula, 72
Bladder tumor = cystoma, 70
Bladder, urinary: see cystis, 70;
    also see Ves. ur., 227
Bladder, urinary, suturing of =
    cystorrhaphy, 57
Bladder, urinary, to look in =
    cystoscopy, 53
Blakiston Company, 228; 249
Blast-, 37
-blast, 45
Blastomycosis, 37
Bleb: see bulla; cutaneous vesicle,
    230
Bleeding points, sealing off method:
    see cauterization, 56
Bleeding tendency: see hemophilia,
    68
Bleeding ties: see ligature, 166
Blepharitis, 74; see also under eyes,
    202
Blepharon, 74; 185
Blepharoptosis, 233
Blind gut: see cecum, 103
Blind, half: see hemianopsia, 161
Blindness: see amaurosis, 34

Blindness, color = achromatopsia,
    129
Blindness, mind: see apraxia, 230
Blindness, night: see nyctalopia,
    173; 230; 242
Blindness, partial = meropia, 39;
    169; 230
Blindness, word: see alexia, 137
Blind passages: see cul-de sac, 151
Blister: see vesica, 110; see also
    bulla; cutaneous vesicle, 230
Blister, blood, 230
Blister, fever: see herpes simplex,
    237; also see cold sore, 232
Blood, 145; 164; see -emia, 46;
    haima, 68; 101; 161; 164
Blood, a flow of = hemorrhage, 48
Blood, bad: see syphilis, 229
Blood blister, 230
Blood cell, red = erythrocyte, 35;
    100; also see R.B.C., 224
Blood cells, red, increase in number
    circulating = polycythemia, 101
Blood cells, white, abnormal increase
    of = leukocytosis, 101
Blood cells, white, destructive to =
    leucotoxic, 34
Blood cell, white: see leukocyte, 46;
    also see W.B.C., 227
Blood count, 207
Blood count, complete: see c.b.c., 213
Blood count, differential: see diff.,
    215
Blood cultures: see under special
    examinations, 208
Blood, excess of white cells in =
    leukemia, 34
Blood, expectoration: see hemopty-
    sis, 161
Blood in stool: see hematochezia, 161
Blood in urine: see hematuria, 49;
    161
Blood in vomit = hematemesis, 68
Blood platelets, decrease in number
    of = thrombopenia, 42
Blood poisoning: see septicemia, 230
Blood, potassium in: see kaliemia,
    164
Blood pressure, 145; 213

Bones, spinal = vertebrae, 66

Bone, tail = coccyx, 65

Bony structures, small: see ossicle, 175

Bony union = synarthrosis, 29

Borborygmus, 145; see also under gastrointestinal, 198; also under abdomen, 205

Border: see limbus, 128

Bore, to: see forare, 124

Boring: see tresis, 142

Born before arrival, 212

Born on arrival, 212

Born, to be: see oriri; gnasci, 116

Born with: see congenital, 29; 151

Born with teeth = dentia praecox, 230

Both: see ambi-, 28

Both sides, on: see amphi-; ampho-, 28

Bottom: see cul, 151; also see fundus, 160

Botulism, 77

Bowed: see kyphos, 93; 165

Bowel: see under cystic fibrosis, 107; also see entero, 104; splanchna, 125

Bowel incontinence, 163

Bowel, injection of fluid into, for nourishment = enteroclysis, 46

Bowel, large = colon, 68

Bowel movement: see excrement, 68; also see defecation, 152; also see B.M., 212

Bowel movement, bloody: see hematochezia, 230

Bowel movement of newborn: see meconium, 158

Bowel movement, stones in: see coprolith, 68

Bowel movement, uncontrolled: see incontinence, 163

Bowels, locked: see intestinal obstruction, 240

Bowels, "loose" = diarrhea, 48

Bowleg: see genu varum, 160; 230

Boxers' fracture, 230

B.P., 213

B.P.H., 213

Brace, 6

Brachial, 6

Brachium, 6

Brachy-, 37

Brachycephalic, 37

Brady-, 37; 145

Bradycardia, 37; 145; also see under heart, 204

Bradypnea, 146; also see under lungs, 204

Brain: see encephalon, 73; 123; also see cerebrum, 123

Brain and spinal cord coverings = meninges, 73

Brain, concussion, 126

Brain, contusion of, 126

Brain, covering, inflammation of = meningitis, 73

Brain covering, protrusion of = meningocele, 27

Brain examination = encephalography, 47; E.E.G., 215

Brain fever: see encephalitis or meningitis, 231

Brain, inflammation of = encephalitis, 73; 126; 231

Brain, laceration of, 126

Brain, left side of: see sinistro-cerebral, 36

Brain, "little" = cerebellum, 123

Brain softening = encephalo-malacia, 126

Brain tissue, protrusion of = encephalocele, 126

Brain tumor, 213

Branchial cleft: see under mouth and throat, 203

Branchial vestiges, 103; see also under mouth and throat, 203

Branchion, 103

Break, to: see fracture, 93; 159

Breast, 83; 198; see mamma; mastos, 4; 130; mammary gland, 64; 83

Breastbone = sternum, 87; 91

Breast, removal entirely = radical mastectomy, 51

Breasts, 203

Breast, suspension or fixation of = mastopexy, 64

Breast swelling, due to accumulation of milk = galactedema, 64

C

$\overline{c}$., 213
C., 213
C_1., C_2., 213
Ca., 213
Cachexia, 146
cal., 213
Cal., 213
Calcareous, 44
Calculated date of confinement: see
  C.D.C., 213
Calculi: see lith, 38; 47; biliary cal-
  culi, 107; cholelithiasis, 44; 107;
  coprolith, 68; cholecystolithiasis,
  238; 246
Calculus: see lithos, 140; see also
  under mouth and throat, 202
Calculus formation on walls of
  aorta: see aortolith, 140
Calculus in the salivary duct: see
  sialolith, 183
Calix, 109
Callosities: see callosus, 123; also
  see under extremities, etc., 206
Callosus, 123
Calorie, large, 213
Calorie, small, 213
Campbell, R. F., XI; 62-63; 250
Cancer, 146; see malignant
  neoplasms; carcinoma, 24; 45
Cancerophobia, 234
Canelike: see baktron, 144
Canker sores: see ulcerations of the
  mouth, 231
Canthi, 127
cap., 213
Cap., 213
Capiat, 213
Capillaries, 98
Capillary pulse: see under heart,
  205
Capsula, 213
Capsule: see cap., 213
Capsule, in a = encapsulated, 30
Capsulorrhaphy, 56
Caput, 86; 89
Carbolic acid: see phenol, 231
Carbon dioxide: see CO_2, 214

Carbuncle, 81; see also subcutaneous
  abscess around hair follicles, 231
Carcinoma, 45; see cancer, 146;
  Ca., 213
Carcinomas, 45
Carcinoma, squamous cell: see
  sq. cell ca., 225
Carcinomata, 45
Card, cardia, 7; 67; 145
Cardiac, 43
Cardiac dilatation, 99
Cardiac hypertrophy, 99
Cardio., 213
Cardiologist, 16; 76; 97
Cardiology, 16; also see cardio, 213
Cardiorespiratory, 198
Cardiorrhaphy, 56
Cardiovascular, 76; see C.V., 214
Cardiovascular disease, 14
Cardiovascular-respiratory: see
  C.V.R., 214
Cardiovascular system, 97-100
Cardiovascular system, diseases of,
  98
Caries, 108; 146; see also under
  mouth and throat, 203
Caries of teeth, 108; 146; 247
Caro, 128
Carotid, 72
Carotid gland, 72; 119
Carotis: see carotid, 72
Carpal bones, 84
Carphologia, 147
Carpus, 65
Cartilage = chondros, 65
Cartilage and bone, destructive in-
  flammation of = osteochondritis,
  94
Cartilage, failure to form = achon-
  droplasia, 48
Cartilage graft, 54
Cartilage, lack of development =
  achondroplasia, 65
Cartilage, semilunar: see meniscus,
  86
Caruncle, 128
Caruncle lacrimalis: see caruncle,
  128
Cata-, 29; 129
Catabolism, 29

Charms: see labia minora, 231
Cheek bone = malar, 85 (or upper jaw bone)
Cheilos, 68
Cheiloschisis, 68
Cheir, 65
Cheirospasm, 248
Chemistry of life: see biochemics, 63
Chest: see thorax, 67; 90; 203; see also pectus, 66; 157
Chest noises: see bruit, 146; crepitus, 151; fremitus, 160; râles; rhonchus, 182; stridor, 184
Chest, to look in = thoracoscopy, 53
Chewer: see masseter, 90
Chewing: see masticating, 231
Chezein, 161
CHI₃, 213
Chickenpox, 81; see also under past history, 198
Chief complaint (C.C.), 196; 213
Child: see puer, 118; 180
Childbearing: see
     bipara, 222
     multipara, 33; 47; 117; 171
     nullipara, 117
     -parous, 47
     unipara, 222
Childbed fever: see puerperal fever, 231
Child before birth: see fetus, 115
Childbirth, discharge following = lochia, 71; 167
Chill or cold shiver: see rigor, 182
Chills and fever, 229
Chin: see geneion, 89
Chin, Andy Gump: see micrognathia, 231
Chin, receding or small: see micrognathia, 231
Chir, 65
Chiro, 147
Chiropodalgia, 147
Chiropodist, 66
Chirospasm, 65
Chloasma, 242
Chloasms, 240
Chlor-, 35
Chloroma, 35
Choking sensation: see angina, 139

Cholangitis, 107
Chole, 68; 105; 136
Cholecystitis, 5; 107
Cholecystolithiasis, 238; 246
Cholecystonosositis, 5
Cholecystorrhaphy, 57
Choledochorrhaphy, 57
Cholelithiasis, 44; 107
Cholelithotripsy, 68
Cholera morbus, 231
Chondrodystrophy of ear, traumatic, 231
Chondros, 65
Chorea, 148; 244
Choreia, 148
Chorion, 115
Choroid, 128
chr., 213
Chroma, 34
Chromatophobia, 234
Chromihidrosis, 34
Chronic, 149; also see chr., 213
Chronos, 149
Chyle: see chylos, 68
Chyle in urine = chyluria, 68
Chylos, 68
Chyluria, 68
Chymos, 109
C.I., 214
Cicatrix, 81; 149
-cide, 45
Cilia, 79; see also under eyes, 202
Cimex, 230
Ciner-, 35
Cinerea, 35
Circum-, 29
Circumocular, 29
Cirrh-, 35
Cirrhosis of liver, 35; 107
Cisterna, 123
Cisterna ambiens, 123
Cisterna basalis, 123
Cisterna magna, 123
Clap: see gonorrhea, 231
-clasis, 55
Claudicare, 149
Claudication, 149
Claudication, intermittent: see leg ache, 240
Claustrophobia, 74; 234

Clavicle, 84
Clavicle, under the = subclavian, 30
Clavus, 232
-cle, 45; 175
Cleaning out dirty wounds = debridement, 56
Cleansing: see catharsis, 147
Clear: see lampros, 165
Clearness of voice: see lamprophonia, 165
Cleft: see fissure, 158; and also under mouth and throat, 202
Cleft, branchial: see under mouth and throat, 203
-cleisis, 46
Climacteric, 149; 225; 231
Clinical findings, accessory, 207
Clinical microscopy: see under clinical pathologist, 18
Clinical Pathological Conference: see C.P.C., 214
Clinical physiologist, 35
Clinical physiology, 25
Clinical psychologist, 24
Clinical psychology, 24
Clinical specialism, 13
Clinician, 13; 150
Clinic, outpatient: see O.P.C., 221
Clitoridectomy, 70
Clitoris, 114; see kleitoris, 70
Clitoris, removal of = clitoridectomy, 70
Clonus, 150
Closed: see -atresia, 45; see also occlusion, 173
Closure: see -cleisis, 46
Closure of normal opening: see atresia, 142
Clothlike: see pannus, 176
Clubfoot: see talipes, 2; 66
Clubfoot, congenital, 92
Clubfoot types: see talipes, 2
-clysis, 46
cm., 214
c.m., 214
C.M., 214
C.N., 214
C.N.S., 214
Co-, 29
CO_2, 214

Coal: see anthrax, 77; 140
Coal dust in lungs: see anthracosis, 140
-coccus (plural = cocci), 46
Coccygeal, 213
Coccygodynia, 65
Coccyx, 65
Coccyx, pain in = coccygodynia, 65
Cochlea, 130
Coition, 150; 232
Cold: see cry-, 37; rigor, 182
Cold, common, 232
Cold in the head: see coryza, 231
Cold, June: see hay fever, 232
Cold (like ice): see crym-, 37
Colds: see under nose and throat, 198
Cold sore: see herpes simplex, 232
Cold, treatment by = crymotherapy, 37
Colic, 150
Colic, renal: see under genitourinary, 199
Colitis, 107
Colon, 68; 103
Colonic, 68
Colon, inflammation of = colitis, 107
Colon (large bowel), relating to = colonic, 68
Color: see chroma, 34
Color blindness = achromatopsia, 129; 232
Colored, many = polychromatic, 33
Color index: see C.I., 214
Colorless: see achromia, 232
Colors, being able to distinguish five = pentachromic, 32
Color vision, 227
Colpocele, 70
Colpoperineorrhaphy, 57
Colporrhaphy, 57
Colpos, 70
Com-, 29
Coma, 151; also see under mental status, 207
Comblike: see pectineus, 90
Comedo, 230
Common water: see aqua communis, 211
Compare: see cf., 213

Cutaneous vesicle, 230

Cutis, 4; 64; 80

Cutis anserina, 238

Cutting: see tome, 49

Cutting into = incision, 49

Cutting off, 52

Cutting out, 51; see excision;
-ectomy; removal, 51

C.V., 214

c.v.a., 214

C.V.A., 214

C.V.R., 214

Cx., 214

Cyan-, 35

Cyanosis, 35; 152; 230; also see
under musculoskeletal system, 206

Cyanotic, 230

cyl., 214

Cylindrical lens, 214

-cyst, 46

Cyst, 247

Cyst distended with fluid: see
hygroma, 162

Cystic fibrosis = mucoviscidosis, 107

Cystic fibrosis of lung, 97; see also
under cystic fibrosis or mucoviscidosis, 107

Cystis, 70

Cystitis, acute: see honeymoon appendicitis, 239

Cystoma, 70

Cystorrhaphy, 57

Cystoscopy, 53; see also under special examinations, 208

Cysts: see under mouth and throat,
202

Cysts containing hair, skin, or teeth
= dermoid cysts, 81

Cysts, dermoid, 81

Cysts, mucous, 82

Cysts, sebaceous: see steatoma, 82;
248

Cyt-, 37

-cyte, 46

Cytoid, 37

Cytologist, 18

Cytology, 18

D

D_1; D_2, 214

Dacrocyst, 46; 128

Dacryocystalgia, 74

Dacryon, 74

Dactylogram, 65; 237

Dactylos, 65; 177

D.A.H., 214

Daily: see in. d., 218

Dance: see chorea, 148

Dandruff: see dermatitis seborrheica,
232

Dark: see amaur-, 34

Darkness: see skotos, 182

Davison, Wilbert C., 19

Day, every: see q.d., 223

Day, every other: see alt. dieb., 211

Day, every third: see dieb. tert., 215

Day, four times a: see q.i.d., 223

Days, alternate: see dieb. alt., 215

Day, three times a: see T.I.D., 226

Day to day: see de d. in d., 214

Day, twice a: see b.i.d., 212

D. & C., 214

D. Cx., 214

D.D., 214

D.D.S., 23

De-, 28; 151

Dead bodies, one who violates =
necrophile, 74

Dead bone: see sequestrum, 232

Dead on arrival: see D.O.A., 215

death: see symbol †, 228

Death, after = postmortem, 31; 222

Death, at the point of: see in
extremis, 218

Debility: see cachexia, 146

Debridement, 56

Deca-, 33

Decanormal, 33

Decayed: see sapro-, 40; 182

Deci-, 33

Decigram, 33

Decompression, 50

Decompression sickness: see
anoxemia, 230

Decub., 214

Decubitus, 152; 214

Decubitus ulcer, 81; 230
Decumbere, 152
De die in diem, 214
De d. in d., 214
Defecation, 152
Definitions, 75
Deflect, 28
Deformities: see under musculo-
skeletal system, 206
Deg., 215
Degeneration: see under deg., 215
Deglut., 215
Deglutiatur, 215
Deglutition, 152
Degree, 215; see also symbol °, 228
Degrees, having one hundred =
centigrade, 33
Dehydration, 152
Delicate: see leptos, 124
Delirium, 242
Delirium tremens, 77
Delivery, before = antepartum, 28
Delivery, breech: see breech presen-
tation of fetus, 118; 146; also see
hind baby, 239
Delivery of child, act of: see
parturition, 177
Deltoideus, 89
Delusions: see under mental status,
207
Dementia, 73
Dementia praecox, 77
Demi-, 33
Demilune, 33
Demonophobia, 235
Demos, 156
Dens, 136; 155
Dental caries, 108
Dental surgeon, 23
Dental surgery, 24
Dentia praecox, 230
Dentist, 23
Dentistry, 24
Dentures, 233; 246; see also under
mouth and throat, 203
Department of Public Dispensary:
see D.P.D., 215
Depressed areas on body: see fossa,
159

Depression: see under mental
status, 207
Depressive, 77
De R., 215
Derm., 215
Derma., 4; 64; 79; 165; 166; 191
Dermatitis, 4; 247
Dermatitis seborrheica, 232; see also
under mange, 241
Dermatologist, 15; 79
Dermatology, 13; 15; see Derm.,
215
Dermatology and syphilology, 15
Dermatophyte, 47
Dermatophytosis, 81; 229
Dermis: see corium, 79
Dermographia: see wheal, 248
Dermoid cysts, 81
Descensus uteri, 233
-desis, 54; 55
Desmo, 65
Desmotomy, 65
Desquamation, 152; 245
Destroy, to: see -clasis, 55
Destruction by electricity: see
fulguration, 56
Destruction, operative procedures of,
55
Destructive reaction: see catabo-
lism, 29
Detached, 52
Detached from: see ablation, 52
Det. in dup., 215
Detur in duplo, 215
Deviation: see under mouth and
throat, 202
Dextro-, 36
Dextrocardia, 36; 99
Di-, 29; 32; 89; 153
Dia-, 29; 56; 84; 152
Diabetes insipidus, 121
Diabetes mellitus, 23; 121; 246
Diabetes, sweet or sugar: see
diabetes mellitus, 246
Diabetic specialist, 23
Diagnoses, provisional, 207
Diagnosis, 152; see Dx, 215
Diagnosis, primary, 208
Diagnostic Roentgenologist, 22
Diaphoreo, 64

Diaphoresis, 152
Diaphoretic, 64
Diaphragm, 65; 66
Diaphragma, 65; 89
Diaphragm and ribs, pertaining to = phrenocostal, 66
Diaphragmatic hernia, 65
Diaphragm, region of, 241
Diaphysis, 84; 86
Diarrhea, 48; 237; also see cholera morbus, 231
Diarrhea with blood content, 230
Diarthrosis, 29
Diastasis recti: see under abdomen, 205
Diathermy, 29; 56
Dicephalous, 65
Dicephalus, 32
Diction: see lexis, 153
Didymoi, 70
Didymos, 111
Dieb. alt., 215
Diebetician, 23
Dieb. tert., 215
Diebus alternis, 215
Diebus tertiis, 215
diff., 215
Different: see hetero-, 38
Differential blood count, 207; 215
Difficult: see dys-, 48; 69; 93; 116; 121; 153; 154
Diffuse, 153
Digastricus, 89
Digestible, 43
Digestive, 102
Digestive system, 68; 102-108
Digestive system, anatomical parts, 102-106
Digestive system, diseases of, 106-108
Digestive tract: see alimentary tract, 102
Digitus, 89
dil., 215
Dilatation: see -ectasia, 58; 96; aneurysm, 138
Dilation and curettage: see D. & C., 214; also see curettage of uterus, 51
Dilute: see dil., 215

Dilutus, 215
Dim: see ambly-, 37
Dim., 215
Diminutive endings: see -ium; -olus; -olum; -culus; -culum; -cle; -cule, 44; 45
Dimness of vision: see amblyopia, 138
Dimness of vision, due to disuse = amblyopia ex anopsia, 73
Dimness of visual acuity: see glimmer, 238
Dimple, chin: see symphysis menti, 232
Diphtheria, 215
Diphtheria bacillus: see K.L. bac., 218
Diphtheria toxin normal, 215
Diplegia, 153
Diplopia, 47; also see under eyes, 198
Dipsa, 68
Dipsomania, 47; 68
Directory of Medical Specialists, XI; 13; 250
Dis-, 153
Disarticulation, 29; 52
Discharge: see under genitalia — male, 205; and also under genitalia — female, 206
Discharge, excessive, from sebacious glands: see seborrhea, 182
Discharge, urethral: see under genitourinary, 199
Discharge, vaginal: see under genitourinary, 199
Discissions, 50
Discoloration, nonelevated: see macule, 82
Discoloration, white, of nails: see leukonychia, 166
Discomfort or distress, vague: see general malaise, 232
Disease: see nosos, 5; -ago; -igo, 45; -pathy, 47; pathos, 73; 162; 168; lesion, 166
Disease, aftereffects: see sequelae, 233
Disease, approach or beginning of: see prodromal stage, 233

Dorsum, 85; 153
Double: see di, 89
Double convex, 214
Double vibrations, 215
Down: see cata-, 28; 129
D.P.D., 215
dr., 215
Drachma, 215
Drainage: see exudate, 157; see also under nose and sinuses, 202
Dram: see dr., 215, and symbol ℨ, 228
Dram, one-sixtieth: see minim, 220
Draw away from = abduct, 135
Drawing spell: see convulsion, epilepsy or hyperventilation, 233
Draw out: see extraction, 51
Draw, to: see ducere, 135; 136
Draw toward, to = adduct, 136
Dread of . . . : see phobias, types of, 234-237
Dread of a beating: see rhabdophobia, 234
Dread of animals: see zoophobia, 234
Dread of assuming responsibility: see hypengyophobia, 236
Dread of becoming a thief or of being kidnapped: see kleptophobia, 236
Dread of bees: see apiphobia, 234
Dread of being fat: see lipophobia, 235
Dread of being touched: see haphephobia, 237
Dread of cancer: see cancerophobia, 234
Dread of childbirth: see tocophobia, 234
Dread of crossing rivers or streams: see potamophobia, 236
Dread of darkness or night: see noctiphobia, 234
Dread of death: see thanatophobia, 234
Dread of eating: see sitophobia, 235
Dread of fever: see febriphobia, 235
Dread of filth: see rhypophobia; rupophobia, 235
Dread of fire: see pyrophobia, 235
Dread of heat or tropics: see thermophobia, 235

Dread of heights: see acrophobia; hypsophobia, 235
Dread of illness: see nosophobia, 235
Dread of lice: see pediculophobia, 235
Dread of lightning: see keraunophobia, 235
Dread of microbes: see microphobia, 235
Dread of moisture: see hygrophobia, 235
Dread of multiple things: see polyphobia, 237
Dread of new things: see neophobia, 235
Dread of pain: see algophobia, 236
Dread of parasites: see parasitophobia, 236
Dread of poisons: see toxicophobia, 236
Dread of riding in trains: see siderodromophobia, 237
Dread of snakes: see ophidiophobia, 236
Dread of stinging insects: see melissophobia, 235
Dread of strangers: see xenophobia, 236
Dread of the sight of blood: see hemaphobia, 234
Dread of tuberculosis: see phthisiophobia, 237
Dread of venereal infection: see venereophobia, 237
Dread of work or being fatigued: see ponophobia, 237
Dreens: see leucorrhea, 233
Dregs: see faex, 152; 158
Dried up: see skeletos, 84
Drink: see bib., 212
Drink, safe to: see potable, 43
Driver's elbow: see bursitis of olecranon, 233
Dromos, 185
Drooping: see -ptosis, 48; 180
Droopy lids: see blepharoptosis, 233
Drop, a: see stranx, 184; also see gt., 217
Drop by drop of urine: see strangury, 184
Dropped womb: see descensus uteri, 233

Drops: see gtt., 217

Dropsy: see edema, 155; 197; 223; 246; see also anasarca; hydrops ascites, 233

Drumlike: see tympanum, 131

Dry: see kraurosis, 165; xeros, 191; xerosis, 191

Dry dressing, 214

Dryness: see xerosis, 191

Dry rot: see caries, 146

Dry skin: see xeroderma, 191

D.S.C., 215

D.T.D., 215

D.T.N., 215

Duct, 103

Duct, lacrimal, 128

Duke University School of Medicine, 133

Dull: see amblys, 138

Dullness, left border of: see L.B.D., 219

Dullness, relative hepatic: see R.H.D., 224

Dullness, submanubrial: see S.M.D., 225

Duodenal ulcer: see peptic ulcer, 108

Duodeni, 103

Duodenorrhaphy, 57

Duodenum, 103

Duodenum, suturing of = duodenorrhaphy, 57

Dura, 123

Dura mater, 123

Dura mater, inflammation of = pachymeningitis, 127

Duration, long: see chronic, 149

Dur. dolor, 215

Dust: see conis, 178

d.v., 215

Dwarf: see nanus, 171

Dwarfish: see nanoid, 171

Dx. (d.x.), 215

Dying condition: see moribund condition, 233

-dynia, 46

Dys-, 48; 69; 96; 116; 121; 153; 154

Dyschondroplasia, 93

Dysentery, 237

Dysentery with bloody content, 230

Dyskinesia, 153

Dyslalia, 153; 245

Dyslexia, 153; 244

Dysmenorrhea, 116; see also under menstrual, 199

Dyspareunia, 153

Dyspepsia, 233

Dysphagia, 69; 154; see also under gastrointestinal, 198; and under mouth and throat, 203

Dysphemia, 154

Dysphonia, 154; see also under mouth and throat, 203

Dysplasia, 153

Dyspnea, 48; 154; 197; see also under cystic fibrosis, 107; also under cardiorespiratory, 198; and under lungs, 204

Dystocia, 154; 240

Dystrophia adiposogenitalis, 121

Dystrophia myotonia congenita, 93

Dystrophy, 48

E

E-, 29; 155; 156

Each eye: see O.U., 221

E.A.H.F., 215

-eal, 43

Ear: see aural, 9; otos, 74; 105; 174; 175; auris, 89; 130; auri, 130; ear, 198

Earache: see otalgia, 131; 233

Ear, bealing in: see otitis media, 229

Ear, broken cartilage with effusion or cauliflower ear: see chondro-dystrophy of ear, traumatic, 231

Ear, draining: see otorrhea, 175

Eardrum: see myringa; tympanic membrane, 74; 131

Eardrum, incision into or puncture = myringotomy, 74

Ear, external, to look in = otoscopy, 53

Ear, fungus of: see otomycosis, 175

Ear, inflammation of = otitis, 74; 131

Ear, left: see auris sinistra, 212

Early in the morning: see mane primo, 219

Ear, nose and throat: see E.N.T., 216

Ear, right: see auris dextra, 210

Ear, rising in: see otitis media, 244

Ears, ringing in = tinnitus, 132; 187; 244

Ear stopped up after flight: see aerotitis, 233

Earthworm-like: see lumbricus, 90

Earwax: see cerumen, 147; 233; 247

Easy: see eu-, 157

Eating: see phagia, 154; 160

Eating earth: see geophagia, 160; 233

Eating rapidly: see tachyphagia, 233

Eating starch: see pica, 233

Eat, to: see phagein, 136; 171; 186

Ec-, 29; 155

Ecchymosis about eyelid, 230

ecg., 215

Echein, 110

Eclampsia, 155

Ect-, 29

E.C.T., 215

-ectasia, 46; 58

-ectasis, 46; 96

-ectomy, 51

Ectonuclear, 29

Ectopic, 155

Ectopic pregnancy, 116

Ectropic, 99

Ectropion, 129; 155; also see under eyes, 202

Eczema, 29; 241; see also under allergic tendencies, 197

Eczema, allergy, hay fever, 215

E.D.C., 215

Edema, 155; 197; 246; see also dropsy, 233; see also under cardio-respiratory, 198; under eyes, 202; under face, 202; and under mouth and throat, 203

Edema, decrease in: see swage down, 246

Edentulous, 155

E.E.G., 215

E.E.N.T., 216

e.g., 216

Egersis, 247

Egg: see Ov., 221

Egophony: see under lungs, 204

Eight: see octa-, 32

E.J., 216

EK., 216

E.K.G. = electrocardiogram, 46; 216

Elbow: see ankon, 88

Elbow, depressed area of: see cubital fossa, 159

Elbow jerk, 216

Elbow joint: see under funny bone, 238

Electric convulsive treatment, 215

Electrocardiogram (E.K.G.), 46; see also under special examinations, 208; ecg.; EK.; EKG.; Ekg., 216

Electroencephalogram (E.E.G.): see under special examinations, 208; 215

Em-, 30

Em., 216

Emaciare, 155

Emaciation, 155

Embolus, 156; see also under encephalomalacia, 126

Embolus, pulmonary, 156

Embryo: see fetus, 115

-emesis, 46; 68

Emesis, 243; 247

-emia, 46; 164

Emmetropia, 216

Emollient, 156

Emphysema, 97; see also under cystic fibrosis, 107

Empyema, 30

Empyema of pleura, 30

En-, 30; 109; 156

Enarthrosis, 229

Encapsulated, 30

Encephalitis, 73; 126; 231

Encephalitis lethargica, 245

Encephalocele, 126

Encephalography, 47

Encephalomalacia, 126

Encephalon, 73

Encephalopathy, 126

Encephalos, 73

Endemic, 156
Endo-, 7; 27; 30; 101; 115
Endocarditis, 7
Endocarditis, bacterial, 99
Endocarditis, rheumatic, 99
Endocardium, 27
Endocervicitis, 4
Endocranium, 27
Endocrin., 216
Endocrine gland, 119
Endocrine system, 72; 118-122
Endocrine system, anatomical parts of, 118-120
Endocrine system, diseases of, 120-122
Endocrinologist, 19; 118
Endocrinology, 19; 216
Endometrium, 30
Endon, 4
Endoscopists, 18
Endoscopy, 18; 53; see also under special examinations, 208
Endoscopy with combined operations, 53
Enophthalmos, 156; see also eyes, 202
Enough: see q.s., 223
Ensiform, 46
Ensiform process, 87
E.N.T., 216
Enteric fever, 69
Enteritis, 108
Enterocleisis, 46
Enteroclysis, 46
Enterolysis, 55
Enteron, 69; 104
Enterorrhaphy, 57
Enterostomy, 55
Ento-, 30
Entocyte, 30
Entrance: see introitus, 163
Entropion, 129; 156; also see under eyes, 202
Enucleate, 29
Enucleation, 51
Enuresis, 156; 230; see also under genitourinary, 199
E.O.M., 216
-eous, 44
Ependyma, 124

Ephelis, 238
Epi-, 30; 79; 85; 111; 156
Epicondyle, 30
Epidemic, 156
Epidemic parotitis, 242; see also under past history, 197
Epidemic pertussis, 248
Epidemiologist, 24
Epidemiology, 24
Epidermis, 64; 79
Epididymis: (didymoi), 70; 111; see also under genitalia — male, 205
Epididymis, cutting the = epididymotomy, 70
Epididymotomy, 70
Epilation, 52
Epilepsy, 73; see also under drawing spell, 233
Epileptiform, 4
Epileptos, 4
Epiphysis, 85; 86
Epiphysis, slipped, 94
Epiplocele, 63
Epiploon, 63
Episioperineorrhaphy, 57
Episiorrhaphy, 57
Epistaxis, 48; 97; 242; also see under nose and throat, 198; also under nose and sinuses, 202
Epulis, 238
Equal: see equi-, 33; is-, 38
Equal parts, in: see P. ae., 222
Equi-, 33
Equilibratory sense, vestibular, 131
Equilibrium, 33
Equina, 123
-er, 44
Erotophobia, 236
Errare, 135
Ertz, Susan, 10; 249
Eructare, 157
Eructation, 157; 197; 230
Eruptions: see under mouth and throat, 202; and also under skin, 201
Erysipelas, 237
Erythroblast, 100
Erythrocyte, 35; 100
Erythrocyte sedimentation rate, 216

Erythropoietic tissue, 100
Erythros-, 35; 100
Eso-, 30
Esophagoptosis, 69
Esophagoscopy, 53
Esophagus, 69; 103
Esophagus, diverticulum of, 108
Esophagus, falling of =
    esophagoptosis, 69
Esophagus, stenosis of, 108
Esophagus, to look in =
    esophagoscopy, 53
Esotropia, 30
E.S.R., 216
-esthesia, 46; 138
Estimated (or expected) date of
    confinement, 215
Estop, 1
Ethmoid bone, 85
Ethmos, 85
Ethnics, 157
Ethnology: see ethnics, 157
Etiol., 216
Etiology, 5; 157; see etiol., 216
Eu-, 157
Euphoria, 244; see also under
    mental status, 207
Eupnea, 157
-eurys, 138
Eustachian tube, 130
Eustachio, Bartolommeo, 130
Even: see homalos, 139
Evening, tomorrow: see cras
    vespere, 214
Everted: see ectropic, 49
Every day: see q.d., 223
Every hour: see omn. hor., 221;
    also see q.h. and q.q. hor., 223
Every night: see omn. noct., 221;
    also see q.n., 223
Every other day: see alt. dieb., 211
Every other hour: see alt. hor., 211
Every other night: see alt. noct., 211
Every third day: see dieb. tert., 215
Evisceration, 52
Ex-, 29; 157
Examination by naked eye: see gross
    or macroscopic examination, 19
Examination, physical, 200

Examinations, spinal fluid: see
    under venereal, 199
Examiner, 44
Excess of: see ultra-, 31; hyper, 34;
    162
Excision, 51
Excision, radical, 51
Excite, to: see hormaein, 161
Excoriated buttocks, 244
Excoriation, 81
Excrement: see copros, 68; feces,
    158
Excrement with stones: see
    coprolith; fecalith, 68
Exempli gratia, 216
Exercise sample no. I, 192
Exercise sample no. II, 193
-exeresis, 51; 52
Exhale, 29
Exia, 181
Exo-, 30
Exogenous, 30
Exophthalmos, 157; see also eyes,
    202
Expansion: see -ectasia; -ectasis, 46
Expected (or estimated) date of
    confinement: see E.D.C., 215
Expecting, 233
Expectoration, 157; 245
Expectoration of blood: see
    hemoptysis 161
Expectoration of pus: see pyoptysis,
    180
Expeller, 46
Exploratory laparotomy, 50
Expression: see under mental
    status, 207
Exstrophy of bladder, 112
ext., 216
Externus, 91
Externus ani sphincter, 91
ext. fl., 216
Extirpation, 51
Extra-, 4; 30; 34
Extract: see ext., 216
Extraction, 51
Extractum, 216
Extraocular movements: see
    E.O.M., 216
Extrasystole, 4; 34

F

Farsightedness = hypermetropia, 129; 234

Fascia, 89

Fascia and muscle sheaths, inflammation of = fibrositis, 93

Fascia, muscles and tendons, 88-92

Fascia, suturing of = fasciorrhaphy, 56

Fasciorrhaphy, 56

Fascist, 89

Fast (speed): see tachy, 40; 186

Fat: see adipose, 44; 136; 234; also see adeps, 121; lipos, 167; steatos, 183

Fat graft, 54

Fauces, 157

Faucial pillars: see under mouth and throat, 203

F.B. (f.b.), 216

F.D., 216

Fear: see phobos, 74

Fear of . . . : see phobias, types of, 234-237

Fear of baldness: see peladophobia, 234

Fear of being near water: see gephyrophobia, 234

Fear of cats: see ailurophobia; galeophobia; gatophobia, 234

Fear of children: see pedophobia, 234

Fear of confined spaces = claustrophobia, 74

Fear of crowds: see koinoniphobia, 234

Fear of doctors: see iatrophobia, 235

Fear of dogs: see kynophobia, 235

Fear of hell: see hadephobia, 235

Fear of lunatics: see demonophobia, 235

Fear of old age: see gerontophobia, 234

Fear of one's own phobias: see phobophobia, 236

Fear of open spaces: see agoraphobia, 236

Fear of poverty: see peniaphobia, 236

Fear of syphilis: see syphilophobia, 236

Fear of talking on the phone: see telephonophobia, 236

Fear of the number 13: see triskaidekaphobia, 236

Fear of the wrath of God: see theophobia, 235

Fear of things on left side = levophobia, 36

Fear of walking on a bridge: see gephyrophobia, 234

Fears, special: see under neuropsychiatric, 199

Febrile, 157; 237

Febriphobia, 235

Febris, 157

Fecal matter containing stones: see coprolith; fecalith, 68

Feces, 158; see also under rectum, 205; and also under special examinations, 208

Feces of newborn: see meconium, 158

Feeling: see -esthesia, 138

Feeling, absence of: see analgesia, 138; anesthesia, 138

Feeling fetal life, 243

Feeling life: see first fetal movement, 237; also quickening, 243

Feel, to: see palpare, 176

Feet, pain in hands and: see chiropodalgia, 147

Fellow of American College of Surgeons, 216

Felon, bone: see osteomyelitis of tip of finger, 230

female: see symbol ♀ or ○, 228

Female, egg-producing organ of: see ovary, 71

Female genitalia, 206

Female genital organs, 114-115

Female genital system, anatomical parts, 114-115

Female genital system, diseases of, 116-118

Female, white: see W.F., 227

Femur, 85

Fencelike: see phragma, 89

Fetal head, engagement of: see lightening, 240

Fetal heart sounds: see F.H.S. (f.h.s.), 216

Fetal movement, first: see feeling life, 237

Fetal structures, 115

Fetor oris, 231

Fetus, 115; 158; 229

Fetus, membrane enclosing = amnion, 115

Fetus, types of presentation, 117-118

Fever: see febris, 157; pyr, 181; pyrexia, 237

Fever blister: see herpes simplex, 237

Fever, cat: see upper respiratory infection, acute, 231

Fever, changing, during a disease: see amphibolia, 138

Fever, childbed: see puerperal septicemia, 231

Fever, childbirth: see puerperal endometritis or metritis, 237

Feverish: see febrile, 157

Fever, parrot: see psittacosis, 242

Fever, rabbit: see tularemia, 244

Fever, rat bite: see sokosha, 244

Fever, red: see erysipelas, 237

Fever, Rocky Mountain spotted: see tick fever, 247

Fever, snail: see schistosomiasis, 237

Fever, swamp or marsh: see malaria, 237

Fever, sweat: see miliaria, 237

Fever, tick: see Rocky Mountain spotted fever, 247

Few: see olig-, 39

F.H., 216

F.H.S., 216

Fibr-, 37

Fibroma, 37

Fibrosis, cystic, of lung, 97; see also under systic fibrosis, 107

Fibrositis, 93

Fibula = see perone, 66; 85

Field of vision: see V.f., 227

Field, per high-power: see /HPF, 218

Fill up, to: see infarcire, 163

Final clinical impressions, 208

Findings, accessory clinical, 207

Finger: see dactylos, 65; 177; digitus/digit, 89

Finger bones = phalanges, 86

Fingerbreadth: see F.B. (f.b.), 216

Fingernail, avulsion of, 51

Fingerprint: see dactylogram, 65; 237

Fingers, too many: see polydactylism, 65 or supernumerary fingers, 34

First: see proto-, 40; 179; primus, 179

Fishbein, Morris, 228; 249

Fissura, 158

Fissure, 81; 158; also see under mouth and throat, 202; and under rectum, 205

Fistula, 97; 158; see also under mouth and throat, 202; and under rectum, 205

Fits: see convulsions, 237

Five: see quinque-, 32; penta-, 32; 177

Five fingers: see pentadactyl, 177

Fixed (stationary): see theto, 142

Fixing in place (fixation or suspension): see -pexy, 54

Fl. (fld.), 216

Flabby: see flaccidus, 158

Flaccid, 44; 158

Flaccidity: see under neurological survey, 206

Flaccidus, 158

Flail chest: see under thorax, 203

Flank: see lapara, 50

Flash out or shine: see lampo, 155

Flat foot, 237, 245

Flat plate: see F.P., 216

Flatulence or flatus, 158; 233; 238

Flatus or flatulence, 158; 233; 238

fl. dr., 216

Flea bites: see pulicosis; pulex irritans, 237

Flectere, 89

Flesh: see sarc(o), 40; sarc, 63; pulpa, 86; kreas (creas), 105

Fleshlike: see caro, 128

Flesh, resembling: see sarcoid, 63

Flexor carpi ulnaris, 89

Flexor digitorum sublimis, 89
F.L.K., 216
Floating kidney: see nephroptosis, 237
Flooding: see menorrhagia, 237
Flow, a: see (r) rhea, 48; 175; see also rhoia, 182, 188
Fl. oz., 216
Fluid: see F. (fl.), 216
Fluid dram, 216
Fluid extract: see ext. flu., 216
Fluid ounce, 216
Fluidum, 216
fluor., 216
Fluoroscopy: see fluor., 216
Fluttering condition: see palpitation, 176
Flux: see diarrhea or dysentery, 237
Flux, bloody: see bloody diarrhea, 230
Focal distance, 216
Foci of infection, 158
Focus, 158
Follicle, 79
Follicle-stimulating hormone: see F.S.H., 217
Follower: see sequela, 183
Food, craving for one kind of: see monophagia, 171
Food, microorganisms in = botulism, 77
Food, unusual craving for: see pica, 178
Foot: see pes, 2; 66; pous, 147; 178; pod, 66
Foot, (12 inches), 217
Foot, flat: see pes valgoplanus, 237
Footprint: see vestigium, 190
Foramen, 124
Force and rhythm of pulse, 216
Forearm bones = radius, 86; ulna, 88
Forecasting outcome = prognosis, 28; 63; 73
Forefoot varus, 243
Foreskin: see prepuce, 111; 237
Foretelling outcome: see prognosis, 179
For example: see e.g., 216

Forgetfulness: see lethargy, 166; lethe, 166
Fork: see -furca, 145
Forked, two: see bifurcation, 145
Form, 46; see morph-, 39; plasis, 154
Forma, 4
Formation: see -plasia, 48
Formed, ill or undeveloped: see dysplasia, 154
Formed, not: see aplasia, 141
Forming: see plasis, 141
Form (or reform): see -plasty, 54
Fornix, 159
Fossa, 159
Fossae, superficial, 79
Fossa, left iliac, 219
Fossa, right iliac, 224
Four: see quadr-; tetra-, 32; 186
Fourchette, 159
Four times a day, 223
Fox: see alopex, 137
F.P., 216
Fracture, boxers': see fracture fifth metacarpal, 231
Fracture of fifth metacarpal, 231
Fractures, 93; 159
Fracture-sprain of distal phalanx, 229
Fractures, types of, 159
Fracturing and refracturing = osteoclasis, 55
Fragrant, 238
Framework-like: see tarsos, 129
Freckle: see ephelis, 238
Free, to: see -lysis, 55
Fremitus, 160; also see under lungs, 204
Fremitus, vocal: see V.F., 227; see also under noise in index
Frenzy: see mania, 77
Friedman test for pregnancy: see Fried., 216
Fried. Test, 216
Fröhlich's syndrome, 121
From (apart): see di-; dis-, 29
From (away from): see ab-; apo-; de-, 28; 116; ab-, 135
From day to day: see de d. in d., 214
From (detached): see ablation, 52

From (out) : see e-; ec-; ex-, 29

Front, near the middle: see antero-median, 36

Front of, in: see antero-, 36

F.S.H. (FSH), 216

ft., 217

-fuge, 46

Fulguration, 56

Fundere, 153

Fundus, 160

Fungus, 82; see myc-, 39; mykes, 174; 175; -phyte, 47

Fungus growth, fleshy = sarcomyces, 40

Fungus infection, 240

Fungus infestation = blastomycosis, 37; 39

Fungus of skin: see under dermatophyte, 47

Fungus of the ear: see otomycosis, 175

Fungus of the nail: see onychomycosis, 174

Funnel chest: see under thorax, 203

Funny bone, 238

Funnygrams, medical: see medical terms, errors in interpretation of, 238

Funny looking kid: see F.L.K., 216

-furca, 145

Furuncle, 81; 230; 243; see also under nose and sinuses, 202

Furunculosis, 230

Fusion, 55

G

Gait and associated movements, 206

Gala, 64

Galactedema, 64

Galactorrhea: see under breasts, 203

Galeophobia, 234

Gallbladder: see G.B., 217; prefix is cholecyst-.

Gallbladder, gravel in: see cholecystolithiasis, 238

Gallbladder, inflammation of: see cholecystitis, 107

Gallbladder, stones in, 246; also see gallstone, 68

Gallbladder, suturing of = cholecystorrhaphy, 57

Galloping consumption: see miliary tuberculosis, 238

Gallstone: see cholelith, 68

Gallstone crushing = cholelithotripsy, 68

Ganglia, spinal, 73

Ganglion, 73; 124

Gangrene, 81

Gas gangrene infection, 81

Gas, oxygen and ether anesthesia: see G.O.E., 217

Gasserian ganglion, 124

Gaster, 4; 69

Gastrectasia, 58

Gastrectomy, subtotal, 51

Gastric disorder or impairment, 233

Gastric ulcer: see peptic ulcer, 108

Gastritis, 4

Gastritis, acute, 106

Gastrocnemius, 89

Gastroenterologist, 15; 16; 102

Gastroenterology, 14; 16; see G.E., 217

Gastroenterostomy, 55

Gastrointestinal, 198; see also G.I., 217

Gastroptosis, 48; 108

Gastrorrhaphy, 57

Gastrorrhexis, 48

Gastroscopy, 53; 69

Gatophobia, 234

G.B., 217

GC., 217

Ge, 160

G.E., 217

Gemellus, 89

Gemellus superior, 89

Geneion, 89

General and special practices in medicine, 12-25

Generalized: see gen'l., 217

Generalized glandular enlargement: see G.G.E., 217

General paralysis of the insane: see G.P.I., 217

General paresis: see G.P., 217

General practitioner, 217

General statement in medical record, 201

H

h., 217

Habit spasm: see tic, 187; 245

Hadephobia, 235

Hag, 246

Haima, 68; 161

Hair, 201; see also pilus, 6; 64; 98; see also trichos, 64; 167; 188

Hair, brittle = trichatrophia, 64

Haircut: see penile chancre, 238

Hair, dry: see xerasia, 238

Hair, falling: see lipsotrichia, 167; 238

Hair follicle: see follicle, 79

Hair, graying: see poliothrix, 238

Hair of head: see capilli, 98

Hair, pulled out by root = epilation of, 52

Hair, rapid loss of: see trichorrhea, 188; 238

Hairy: see hirsutism, 161; hirsute, 201; 238; pilous, 64

Half: see demi-, 33; hemi-, 33; 161; semi-, 33; 131

Hallucinations, 161; see also under mental status, 207

Hallucinosis, 77

Hallux valgus, 231; see also under musculoskeletal system, 206

Hamlike or back of knee: see popliteus, 90

Hammertoe, 238

Hamstring, 239

Hand: see cheir; chir, 65; 147

Handling: see manipulation, 58

Hand, part between wrist and fingers = metacarpal region, 65

Hands, able to use both well = ambidextrous, 28

Hands and feet, pain in: see chiropodalgia, 147

Hands and feet, slow involuntary movement of: see athetosis, 142

Hangnail, infected: see paronychia, 82; 239

Haphephobia, 237

Hard: see scirrho-; sclero-, 40; see also under dura, 123; and under sclera-, 129

Hardening = sclerosing, 40

Hard-skinned = callosus, 123

Harelip = cheiloschisis, 68; see also under congenital, 151; and under mouth and throat, 202

Hawking and snorting: see screatus, 239

Hay fever: see allergic rhinitis, 239; see also cold, June, 232

Hb., 217

HCL., 217

H.C.V.D., 217

H.d., 217

H.D., 217

Head, 198; 201; see cephale, 65; 147; 162; see also caput, 86; 89

Headache: see cephalalgia, 147

Headache on both sides = amphicrania, 28

Headache, sick: see migraine, 239

Head bone, at back = occipital, 86

Head, cold in the: see coryza, 231

Head, long = dolichocephalous, 37

Head, pointed = oxycephalic, 39; 243

Head presentations of fetus, 117

Head, short = brachycephalic, 37

Heads, two = dicephalous, 65

Head, water: see hydrocephalus, 247

Head, wide = platycephalic, 39

Health, ill: see cachexia, 146

Hearing distance, 217

Hearing, sense of = acoustic sense, 127; 130-132

Heart, 204; see also cardia, 7; 67; 145; cor, 178

Heart, anomaly, having four features of = Tetralogy of Fallot, 32

Heart arteries, narrowing of = stenocardia, 40

Heart attack: see coronary artery occlusion, usually, 239

Heartbeat, fast = tachycardia, 40

Heartbeat, slow: see bradycardia, 37; 145

Heartburn, 239

Heart chamber: see ventricle, 98

Heart contraction, additional = extrasystole, 34

Ligare, 90
Ligatura, 166
Ligature, 166
Light: see phot-, 39
Light and accommodation: see
  L. & A. (l/a), 219
Lightening, 240
Light, fear of (intolerance to) =
  photophobia, 39
Light perception, 222
Light, to: see illuminare, 188
Like: see -oid, 47; 91; 101; 102;
  120; 122; 167; 171; 191
Liking: see philia, 74
Limbus, 128
Limosis, 239
Limp, to: see claudication, 149
Line (streak or furrow): see stria,
  184
Linea, 167
Lineae albicantes, 167
Lingua, 69; see under tongue, 106
Lingual lesions: see under
  gastrointestinal, 198
Lingual tonsils, 69; see also under
  mouth and throat, 202
Lining: see endo-, 7; mucous
  membrane, 80
Lining, abdominal = peritoneum, 63
Lining of abdominal and pelvic wall
  = parietal peritoneum, 78-79
Lip: see cheilos, 68; labium, 114;
  165; see also under mouth and
  throat, 202
Lipoid, 167
Lipoids in the skin characterized by
  flat plaque of yellow: see
  xanthoma, 191
Lipophobia, 235
Lipos, 167
Lip reading: see labiology, 165
Lips, large = macrocheilia, 38
Lipsotrichia, 167; 238
Liq., 219
Liquid, 219
Liquid solution, 219
Liquor, 219
Lisping: see dyslalia, 153
Listen, to: see auscultare, 143
Liter: see L. (l.), 219

-lith, 47
Lith-, 38; 183
Lithos, 140
Lithotripsy, 38
Liver, 104; also see hepato, 69;
  see also under abdomen, 205
Liver, atrophy of, 107
Liver biopsies: see under special
  examinations, 208
Liver, cirrhosis of, 35; 107
Liver, congestion, 107
Liver, fixation of = hepatopexy, 69
Liver fluke: see opisthorchis
  viverrini, 240
Liver function test: see Vand., 227
Liver, inflammation of: see
  hepatitis, 108
Liver secretion = bile, 103
Liver, spleen and kidneys: see
  L.S.K., 219
Liver spots: see chloasms, 240
Liver, suturing of = hepator-
  rhaphy, 57
Living and well: see L. & W., 219
L.L., 219
L.L.Q., 219
L.M.A., 118
L.M.D., 12; 219
L.M.P., 118; 219
L.O.A., 117; 219
Lobar pneumonia, 97
Localized, not: see diffuse, 153
Local Medical Doctor = L.M.D.,
  12; 219
Lochia, 71; 167
Lochia, excessive flow of =
  lochiorrhagia, 71
Lochiorrhagia, 71
Lochios, 71; 167
Locked bowels: see intestinal
  obstruction, 240
Lockjaw: see tetanus, 78; 188; 241
-logia, 147; 166
Logorrhea, 246
Logos = study of, 76; 157; 165
-logy, 47
Loin: see psoa, 91
Long: see dolicho-, 37
Long duration: see chronic, 149

M

Melos, 169

Membrane: see meninges, 73; 124; also see under mucosa, 80 or mucous membrane, 80; also tympanic membrane under ears, 201

Memory: see mnesis, 73

Memory, defective: see under neuropsychiatric, 199

Memory, loss of = amnesia, 73

Menarche, 116; 169

Ménière's disease, 131

Ménière's syndrome, 185

Meninges, 73; 124

Meningitis, 73; 231

Meningocele, 27

Meninx, 73

Meniscus, 86

Meniscus of jaw, dislocation of: see snapping jaw, 245

Menopause, 116; 231; 247

Menorrhagia, 117; 237

Mens, 73

Menstrual, 199; also see menstruation, 116-117

Menstrual period, last: see L.M.P., 219

Menstrual period, previous: see P.M.P., 223

Menstruation, cessation: see amenorrhea, 116

Menstruation, excessive: see menorrhagia, 117

Menstruation has ceased, 229

Menstruation, natural cessation of: see menopause, 116

Menstruation, onset of = menarche, 116; 169

Menstruation, painful = dysmenorrhea, 116

-ment, 145

Mental age, 219

Mentally slow: see lethargia, 166

Mental state, morbid: see psychosis, 63

Mental state of great calm: see psychodelic, 241

Mental status, 207

Mer-, 39

Mercury: see Hg, 217

Mercury, millimeters of: see mm. Hg, 220

Meropia, 39; 169; 230

Meros, 169

Merriam Company, G. and C., 250

Mesenchyme, 78

Mesenteroid, 69

Mesentery, 69; 104

Mesentery, pertaining to = mesenteroid, 69

Mesos-, 36; 78; 104

Mesos-enteron, 69

Mesosternum, 36

Meta-, 31; 86; 170

Metabolism, 170

Metacarpal, 65

Metacarpal, fracture of fifth: see Boxer's fracture, 231

Metaphysis, 86

Metaplasia, 31

Metastasis, 48; 170

-meter, 47

Meter = 39.37 inches, 33

Meters, one thousand = kilometer, 33

Meter, thousandth part of = millimeter, 33

Metra, 4; 115; 180

Metritis, 237

Metrorrhagia, 48; 117; see also under menstrual, 199; 243; 245

mg., 220

M.H., 220

M.I., 220

Mic., 220

Micro-, 15; 39; 170

Microcephaly, 127

Microcoria, 170; 243

Micrognathia, 170; 231

Microorganisms: see under bacterium, 15; 144

Microphobia, 235

Microscope, 39

Microscopic findings: see Mic., 220

Microscopist, 19

Microscopy, clinical, 19

Micturition, 170

Mid-clavicular line: see M.C.L., 220

Middle of: see medi-; mes-, 36; 78; 104

Midriff: see diaphragm, region of, 241

Mid-sternal line: see M.S.L., 220

Migraine, 10; 239

Miliaria, 237; 243

Miliary, 170

Miliary tuberculosis, 238

Milk: see galact, 64; see also lacteal, 43

Milk crust: see under cradle cap, 232

Milk leg: see phlegmasia alba dolens, 241

Milk rash = eczema, 241

Milky: see lacteal, 43

Milli-, 33

Milligram, 220

Millimeter, 33; see mm., 220

Millimeters of mercury: see mm. Hg, 220

min., 220

Mind: see psyche, 63; mens, 73; soul, 76

Mind blindness: see apraxia, 141; 230

Mind, ill in: see psychopath, 73

Mind, loss of: see dementia, 73

Mindreader: see telepathist, 241

Mind, to wander in: see hallucination, 161

Miner's elbow: see bursitis of olecranon, 241

Miniature: see -ium; -olus; -olum; -culus; -culum; -cle; -cule, 44-45

Minim, 220; also see symbol $\mathcal{M}$, 228

Miscarriage, 241

Misery: see pain, 241

Mishap: see abortion, 241

Mite: see acarus, 135; 241

Mites, infested with: see acariasis, 135

Mitral first sound, 219

Mitral insufficiency, 220

Mitral stenosis, 220

Mitral valve, 98

mix: see m, 228

Mixed astigmatism with exceeding myopia, 211

mm., 220

M.M., 220

mm. Hg, 220

Mnesis, 73

Moist: see hygro, 162

Molding: see plasis, 141

Mole, blue: see nevus pigmentosus, 230

Molecule, 45

Moles: see nevi (pl.) or nevus, 242

Mollis, 156

Mon-, 31; 171

Monilia, 174

Moniliasis, 247

Monocytes, 219

Mononuclear, 31

Monophagia, 171

Monophobia, 234

Montanus, 110

Moon, (half-moon formation): see demilune, 33

Morbid dislike of . . . : see phobias, types of, 234-237

Morbid dislike of air or drafts: see aerophobia, 234

Morbid dislike of being alone: see monophobia, 234

Morbid dislike of closed-in spaces: see claustrophobia, 234

Morbid dislike of dust: see coniophobia, 235

Morbid dislike of sexual love: erotophobia, 236

Morbid dislike of speaking: see lalophobia, 236

Morbid dislike of the male sex: see androphobia, 236

Morbidity, 171

Morbid mental state: see psychosis, 63

Moribund, 171

Moribund condition, 233

Morning, early in the: see Man. pr., 219

Morning sickness: see hyperemesis gravidarum, 242

Morning, tomorrow: see cras mane, 214

Morph-, 39

Morphology, 39

Mortality, 171

Mother: see mater, 123

Motion: see kinesis, 164

N

Noise, rumbling of bowels: see bor-
borygmus, 145
Nolle prosequi, 1
Nolo contendere, 1
Nomos, 123
Nonagenarian, 32
Nonprotein nitrogen tests (N.P.N.),
221
Noon, before: see A.M., 211
Normal temperature and pressure,
221
Nose: see nasus, 175; rhin, 67; 96;
202; also see rhis, 96; 181
Nose and sinuses, 202
Nose and throat, 198
Nosebleed = epistaxis, 48; 97; 242
Nose bone = vomer, 88
Nose stopped up: see hypertrophic
rhinitis, 242
Nose, surgical repair of = rhino-
plasty, 54; 67
Nose, swelling of = rhinophyma, 42
Nose, to look in = rhinoscopy, 53
Nosophobia, 235
Nosos, 5
Nosositis, 5
Nostril: see nares, 95
Not: see an-, 31; 139; 161; in, 163
Nourishment: see troph-, 41; 48;
82; -trophe, 142; 162; 188
Nourishment, faulty = dystrophy,
48
Novem-, 33
Novemlobate, 33
N.P.N., 221
N. Surg., 221
N.T.P., 221
Nucleus, 86
Nucleus pulposus, 86
Nullipara, 117
Nulliparous, 173
Number, 220
Number, too many in = supernu-
merary, 34
Numbness: see narc-, 39; see also
paresthesia, 242
Numero, 220
Nunc pro tunc, 1
Nurse-anesthetist, 14-15
Nv., 221
Nyctalopia, 173; 230; 242
Nyctophobia, 234
Nymphe, 71
Nymphoncus, 71

Nystagmus, 130; 173; also see under eyes, 202

O

$\overline{O}$ = pint, 228
O.B. (Ob.) (Obs.), 221
Obese or obesity, 173; also see fat,
234
O.B.-Gyn., 221
Obliteration, 51
Obstetrician, 16; 114
Obstetrics, 16; also see O.B. (Ob.)
(Obs.), 221
Obstetrics and gynecology, 14; 16-
17; see O.B.-Gyn., 221
Obstruction: see under nose and
sinuses, 202
Obstruction, intestinal: see locked
bowels, 240
Occipital bone, 86
Occlusion, 173
Occlusus, 173
Octa-, 32
Octagonal, 32
Ocular tension: see under eyes, 202
Oculus dexter, 221
Oculus sinister, 221
Oculus uterque, 221
O.D., 17; 221
Odont, 69
Odontodynia, 69
Odor: see under olfactory sense, 127;
see also under menstrual, 199
Odyne, 174
Of: see de, 151
Of each, 210
Of which, 214
-oid, 47; 91; 94; 101; 102; 120;
122; 130; 164; 167; 171; 191
Oidema, 97; 155; 188
Oil, 221
Ointment, 227
Oisophagos, 69
ol., 221
Old: see presbys, 179; senile, 182
Old age: see geras, 137; 179
Old age, appearance of, in child:
see progeria, 179; 229
Old tuberculin: see O.T., 221
Olecranon, 10
Olecranon, bursitis of: see under
driver's elbow, 233; see also
miner's elbow, 241

Olecranon process, 86; also see under funny bone, 238
Oleum, 221
Olfactophobia, 236
Olfactory sense, 127; 198
Olig-, 39
Oligos, 174
Oliguria, 39; 174
Olive oil, 221
ol. oliv., 221
-olum, 44
-olus, 44
-oma (plural = omata), 45; 139; 142; 162; 191
-omata, 45
Omentum, 63; 78
omn. hor., 221
omn. noct. (o.n.), 221
Omodynia, 66; 174
Omos, 66; 174
Omphalos = umbilicus, 79
On alternate days, 215
Onc-, 39
Oncologist, 24
Oncology, 24
Oncotherapy, 174
One: see uni-; mono-, 31
One and one-half hour: see sesquihora, 33
One-half: see Dim., 215; also see ss, 225
One-sixtieth of dram: see min., 220
One's own: see idio-, 38; idios, 162
One versed in: see -ician, 13
One who practices: see -ist, 44; -or; -er; -ician, 44
Onkos, 174
Onset stage of illness, relating to: see prodromal, 43
Onychia, 64
Onychoclasis, 242
Onychomycosis, 174
Onychophagia, 242
Onychophyma, 64
Onyx, 82; 166; 169; 174
O.O.B., 221
Oöphorein, 71
Oöphoropathy, 71
Oophororrhaphy, 57
Opacities, corneal: see under eyes, 202
O.P.C., 221
O.P.D., 221
Open: see patent, 110

Openings: see introitus; meatus; mouth; orifice; os, 242
Open, not: see atresia, 142
Open reduction, 54
Operating room: see O.R., 221
Operational incisions and abdominal regions, 59
Operation, examples of:
    amputation, 52-53
    destruction, 55-56
    endoscopy, 53-54
    esdoscopy with combined procedures, 54
    excision, 51-52
    incision, 49-50
    introduction, 52-53
    manipulation, 58
    repair, 54-55
    suturing, 56-57
    (types of sutures), 57
Operations combined with endoscopy, 54
Operator, 44
Ophidiophobia, 236
Ophth., 221
Ophthalmia, 74
Ophthalmocopia, 174; 233
Ophthalmologist, 17; 127
Ophthalmology, 14; 17; see Ophth., 221
Ophthalmos, 74; 128; 156; 157; 174
Ophthalmoscopic examination: see under eyes, 202
-opia, 47; 138; 139; 169; 173; 179
Opisth-, 36
Opisthen, 174
Opisthorchis viverrini, 240
Opisthotic, 174
Opisthotonos, 36
Opsia, 161
Opsis, 51; 73; 143; 172
Optician, 17
Optic thalamus, 124
Optometrist, 17
-or, 44
O.R., 221
Oral, 9
Oral surgeon, 24
Oral surgery, 24
Orbicularis, 90
Orbicularis oculi, 90
Orbis, 128
Orbit, 128
Orchis, 71
Orchitis, 113

P

Q

R

S

Spitting: see ptysis, 161; 180; also see expectoration, 157; 245

Spitting blood: see hemoptysis, 161; 245

Spitting up: regurgitation, 245

Splanchna, 125

Splanchnic nerve, 125

Splanchnoptosis, 180

Splayfoot: see flatfoot, 245

Spleen, 101; 166; also see splen, 68; also under abdomen, 205

Spleen and kidney: see lienorenal, 166

Spleen, removal of = splenectomy, 68

Splen, 68; 101

Splenectomy, 68

Splenion, 91

Splenius, 91

Split in two: see bifidus, 94

Spondylitis, 66

Spondylitis deformans, 243

Spondylolisthesis, 94

Spondylos, 66; 94

Sport: see playboy, 243

Spot on retina, yellow: see y.s., 228

Spots before eyes: see scotoma, 245

Spotting: see metrorrhagia, 245

Sputum, 184; see also under cardiorespiratory, 198

Sputum examination: see under special examinations, 208

sq. cell ca., 225

Squama, 152

Squamous cell carcinoma, 225

Squinting: see strabismus, 130

S.R., 225

s.s., 225

SS. (ss.), 225

S.S.V., 225

Stabilization, 55

Stafflike: see baktron, 144

Stalsis, 177

Stammering: see dysphemia, 154

Stammers, one who: see R.L.S. person, 224

Standard Nomenclature of Diseases and Operations, XI; 63; 76; 157; 208; 250

Standard nomenclature of operations, 49

Standing: see stasis, 175

Standing upright: see orthostatic, 175

Staph., 225

Staphylococcus: see staph., 225

-stasis, 48; 175

Stat., 225

Statement, general, 201

Statim, 225

-staxis, 48

Stb., 225

STD, 225

Steatoma, 82; 248

Steatopygia, 184; 231

Steatos, 183

Stems, 61-74

  body as a whole, 63

  cardiovascular, 67

  digestive system, 68-70

  endocrine system, 72

  hemic and lymphatic system, 68

  integumentary system, 64

  nervous system, 73-74

  organs of special sense, 74

  respiratory system, 66-67

  urogenital system, 70-72

Sten-, 40; stenos, 97; 184

Stenocardia, 40

Stenosis, 184; 242

Stenosis of esophagus, 108

Step: see basis, 135

Stereo, 40; 225; 245

Stereogram, 225

Stereoscopic, 40

Sternocleidomastoideus, 91

Sternon, 4; 87; 91

Sternum, 87

Sternum, middle part: see gladiolus, 44

Sternum, upper part = manubrium, 44

Sternutation, 184

Sternutation, producing: see quilling, 243

Stertor, 245

Stet., 225

Stethoscope: see under auscultation, 143

-sthen, 48; sthenos, 141

Stiff and crooked: see ankylosis, 139

Stiffening: see spastic, 183

Stillborn, 225

Stoma, 49; 70; 106

Stomach, 4; 69; 106; see also gaster, 4; 69; stomachus, 4; 106

Stomach and intestines, gas or air in: see flatus, 238

Stomach content examination: see under special examinations, 208

Subepithelial hematoma, 230
Sublingual and salivary glands, 202
Submanubrial dullness, 225
Subnormal, 34
Sub signo veneni, 225
Subspecialists, 15-16
Subspecialties, 14
Substernal, 4
Substituting with artificial part: see
    prosthesis, 179
Subtotal or partial removal, 51
Succussion, 185; also see under ab-
    domen, 205
Succutere, 185
Sudare, 157
Sudarium, 246
Sudoresis, 243
Sudoriferous glands, 80
Sudorrhea, 243
Suet: see sebum, 182
Sufficient quantity: see q.s., 223
Suffix, diminutive, 79
Suffixes, 7; 43-58
Suffixes, instruction in, 27; 43
Suffixes, words, and phrases on
    operative terminology, 49
Sug., 226
Sugar, 226
Sugar diabetes, 246
Suggestions (history and physical
    examination), 207
Summary (history and physical
    examination), 207
Sunburn: see actinic dermatitis,
    246
Sunstroke: see heatstroke, 239
Sunstroke or heatstroke: see
    siriasis; thermoplegia, 187; 239
Super-, 31; 34
Superciliary, 31
Supercilium, 233
Superficial fossae, 79
Supernumerary, 34
Supinare, 92
Supinator, 92
Supine position, 241
Suppression, 185
Suppurative nephritis, 113
Supra-, 31
Suprapubic, 31
Suprarenal gland: see adrenal
    gland, 119
Surg., 226
Surgeon, general, 22
Surgeon, oral, 24

Surgeon, orthopedic, 17; 22
Surgeon, plastic, 20; 22
Surgeon, thoracic, 23
Surgery, 14
Surgery, neurological, 14; 16
Surgery, oral, 24
Surgery, plastic, 14; 20; 24
Surgery, surgical or surgeon, 226
Surgery, thoracic, 14; 22; 23
Surgical Chiropody, Doctor of:
    see D.S.C., 215
Surgical postures, 60
Surgical urology, 14; 23
Sutures: see under head, 201
Suturing: see -(r)rhaphy, 56
Suturing material, 57
    catgut; horsehair; silkworm;
    linen; metal clips
Swage down: see decrease in edema,
    246
Swallowing: see phagia; phagein,
    69; 171; 186; deglutition, 152
Swallowing air: see aerophagia,
    136; 229
Swallowing, difficult = dysphagia,
    69
Swallowing, painful: see dysphagia,
    154
Swayback = lordosis, 93; 167; 246;
    also see saddleback, 244
Sweat: see hidrosis, 246; see also
    sudor, 246
Sweat bath: see sudarium, 246
Sweat, colored = chromhidrosis, 34
Sweat glands = sudoriferous
    glands, 80
Sweating, profuse: see hyper-
    hidrosis, 162; perspiration, 243
Sweat, to: see sudare, 157
Sweet or sugar diabetes, 246
Swelling: see -cele, 45; edema, 97;
    155; 246; also oidema, 188
Swelling due to altered nourish-
    ment = trophoedema, 41; 188
Swelling of feet and legs: see
    trophedema, 188
Swelling or mass: see tumor, 189
Swoon: see syncope, 246
Swordlike: see xiphoid, 191
Sword-shaped: see ensiform, 46
Sycosis barbae, 229
Sycosis vulgaris, 229
Sym-, 29; 87
Symblepharon, 185; also see under
    eyes, 202

Symphysis, 29; 87
Symphysis menti, 232
Symphysis pubis, 86
Symptoms occurring together: see
    syndrome, 185
Syn-, 29; 87; 116; 185
Synarthrosis, 29; 64
Syncope, 185; see also under cardio-
    respiratory, 198; 246
Syncytium, 116
Syndactylism, 247; see also under
    musculoskeletal system, 206
Syndrome, 185
Syph., 226
Syphilis, 15; also see lues, 168; 229;
    245
Syphilis, latent, 165
Syphilis microorganism =
    Treponema pallidum, 15
Syphilis, primary lesion = chancre,
    112
Syphilis, serology test for, 226
Syphilis, venereal disease: see
    V.D.S., 227
Syphilitic arthritis, 94
Syphilologist, 15
Syphilology, 15; 226
Syphilophobia, 236
Syphon: see under diabetes, 121
Syr., 226
Syrup, 226
Syrupus, 226
Systole, 4
Systremma, 232

T

T., 226
T&A, 226
T.A.B., 226
Tabacosis, 185
Tabacum, 185
Tabes, 127
Tabes dorsalis, 127
Tachis, 186
Tachy-, 40
Tachycardia, 40; also see under
    heart, 204
Tachycardia, paroxysmal auricular:
    see PAT, 222
Tachyphagia, 186; 233
Tachypnea, 186; also see under
    lungs, 204

Tactile, 186
Tactile fremitus, 226; also see un-
    der noise in index; see also under
    lungs, 204
Tactilis, 186
Tags: see under mouth and throat,
    203
Tail: see cauda, 246
Tail bone: see coccyx, 65
Tailor: see sartor, 91
Talipes, 2; 66
Talipes arcuatus, 2
Talipes calcaneovalgus, 2
Talipes calcaneovarus, 2
Talipes calcaneus, 2
Talipes cavus, 2
Talipes equinovalgus, 2
Talipes equinovarus, 2; 92
Talipes equinus, 2; 92
Talipes percavus, 2
Talipes planus, 2
Talipes valgus, 2; 245
Talipes varus, 2; 92
Talking: see lalia, 153
Talking, excessive: see lalorrhea;
    logorrhea, 246
Talus, 2
Tarsal bones, 88
Tarsus, 129
-tasis, 58
Taste, sense of = gustatory sense,
    127
T.A.T., 226
Tbc (tbc), 226
Tear (tēr), a: see lacrima, 128
Tear (târ) away: see avulsion, 51
Tear (tēr) duct: see dacryocyst, 46;
    dacryon; lacrimal sac, 74
Tear duct, pain in = dacryocystal-
    gia, 74
Tear glands and ducts = lacrimal
    glands and ducts, 128
Teeth: see under gastrointestinal,
    198; see also under mouth and
    throat, 203
Teeth, born with: see dentia
    praecox, 230
Teeth, buck: see protrusion of
    upper incisors, 246
Teeth, caries of = dental caries,
    108; 146; 247
Teeth, decayed = saprodontia, 40;
    dental caries, 108

Teeth, decayed, missing, and filled: see D.M.F., 215

Teeth, false: see dentures, 233

Teeth grinding of: see trismus, 188; bruxism, stridor, dentium, 246

Teeth, large = megadontia, 38

Teeth, store: see dentures, 246

Teeth, widely separated: see hag or rake, 246

Teeth, without: see adentia, 136; edentulous, 155

Teinein, 63; 78

Telalgia, 242

Telangiectasia: see under skin, 201

Telepathist, 241

Telephonophobia, 236

temp. dext., 226

Temperature, 226

Temperature, pulse and respiration, 226

Temple bone = temporal, 88

Temple, right, 226

Temporal bone, 88

Tempus dextra, 226

Ten: see deci-; deca-, 33

Tendencies, allergic, 197

Tendere, 92; 125

Tendon: see tenon, 66; 92; see also under neurological survey, 206

Tendon, cutting a = tenotomy, 66

Tendon, lengthen or shorten, 54

Tendons, attach or reattach, 54

Tendon sheath, inflammation of = tenosynovitis, 95

Tendon, suturing of = tenorrhaphy, 56

Tenesmus, 186; see also under genitourinary, 199

Tennis elbow: see radio-humeral elbow, 247

Tenon, 66

Tenorrhaphy, 56

Tenosynovitis, 95

Tenotomy, 66

Tension, equal: see isotonic, 38

Tensor, 92

Tensor veli palatini, 92

Tentorium, 125

ter-, 32

Teres, 92

Teres major, 92

Ter in die, 226

Terminology, lay, 229-248; also refer to index for word

Tertiary, 32

Testa, 111

Test, complement-fixation: see C.F.T., 213; also see test for syphilis in index

Testes: see under genitalia — male, 205

Test for cancer: Papanicolaou (smear of cervical and vaginal secretions): see under genitalia — female, 206

Test for deafness: Weber's, 210

Test for hearing: Weber's, 210

Test for pregnancy: Ascheim-Zondek, 212 Friedman, 216 Salmon

Test for syphilis: see STS, 226 Cardiolipid titer Eagle Hinton Kahn Kline Kolmer (esp. spinal fluid) Mazzini V.D.R.L. (Venereal Disease Research Laboratory)

Test for tuberculosis: Mantoux

Test for typhoid: Widal

Testicle: see orchis, 71; testis, 111

Testicle, inflammation of = orchitis, 113

Testicles, undescended = cryptorchidism, 37; 71; 112

Testis, 111; also see orchis and testicle, 71; gonads, 119; also see under hydrocele, 45

Testis and ovary: see under gonad, 72; 119

Testis, collection of fluid in = hydrocele, 45

Testis, small body lying above = epididymis, 70

Test, kidney functions: see P.S.P., 223

Test, liver function: see Vand., 227

Test, phenolsulfonphthalein, 208; 223

Test solution, 226

Testum, 111

Tumor, green = chloroma, 35
Tumor of bladder = cystoma, 70
Tumor, smooth muscle = leyo-
myoma, 38
Tumor, treatment of = oncho-
therapy, 39
Tunica, 112
Tunica vaginalis, 45; 112
Turbinates, 96
Turmoil: see clonus, 150
Turn back, to: see reflex, 181
Turned outward = ectropic, 49
Turning, a: see tropic, 49; trope,
155; 156
Turning inward of eyelid: see
entropion, 156
Turning outward of eyelid: see
ectropion, 155
Tus. (tus.), 226
Tussis, 189; 226
Twelve = duodeni, 103
Twice a day: see b.i.d., 212
Twinge: see short, sharp pain, 247
Twinlike: see gemellus, 89
Twisted = tortus, or torsion, 95
Twitching: see tic, 187
Two: see bi-, 32; 89; 145; bin-, 32;
di-, 32; 153
Two-eyed: see binocular, 32
Two-forked: see bifurcation, 145
Two heads = dicephalus, 32
Two sides, affecting: see bilateral, 32
Tympanic membrane = ear drum,
74; 131; see also under ears, 201
Tympanum, 131
Type and rate of breathing: see
under lungs, 204
Typhoid, 47
Typhoid fever: see enteric fever, 69
Typhoid para A and B vaccine, 226

U

U.C.H.D., 226
U.D., 226
Ulcer, 83; 189
Ulcerations: see under nose and
sinuses, 202
Ulcerations of mouth: see under
mouth and throat, 202; 203; 231
Ulcer, decubitus, 81; 152; also see
bedsore, 230
Ulcer, duodenal: see peptic ulcer,
108

Ulcer, gastric: see peptic ulcer, 108
Ulcer, peptic, 108
Ulcer, trophic, 82
Ulcer, varicose, 83
Ulcus, 83; 189
Ulna, 88
Ulna, projection at head of =
coronoid process, 84
Ulnar nerve: see under funny bone,
238
ult., 226
Ultimum, 226
Ultra-, 31
Ultrasterile, 31
Umb., 227
Umbilical cord, 116
Umbilicus, 79; 116; 227; see also
under abdomen, 205
Unborn offspring: see fetus, 115;
158; 229
Unconsciousness: see coma, 151
Under: see infra-; hypo-, 30; sub-,
30; 80
Under a poison label: see S.S.V.,
225
Undersized: see atrophy, 142
Undescended testicles = cryp-
torchidism, 37; 71; 112
Undeveloped or ill-formed: see
dysplasia, 154
Unequal: see aniso, 139
Unequal pupils: see anisocoria, 139
Unequal vision in the two eyes:
see anisopia, 139
Uneven: see scalenus, 91
Ung. (ung.), 227
Unguis incarnatus, 240; see also
under musculoskeletal system, 206
Uni-, 31
Unicellular, 31
Unipara: see Para I, 222
United States Pharmacopoeia, 227
United States Public Health
Service, 227
Unit of X-ray dosage, 228
Up, apart, or across: see ana-, 28
Up-chuck: see emesis, 247
Upon: see epi-, 30; 111; 156
Upper end: see apex, 140
Upper respiratory infection, 227
Upper respiratory infection, acute,
231
Upright position: see orthopnea, 175
Upside-down stomach: see thoracic
stomach, 247

Ur. (ur.), 227
Urachus, 110
Urachus, patent, 110
Uremia: see under anuria, 140
Ureter, 110
Ureteral stricture, 113
Ureterorrhaphy, 57
Ureterovesical, 110
Ureter, suturing of = ureteror-
rhaphy, 57
Urethra, 110
Urethral discharge: see under
genitourinary, 199; 226
Urethral orifice: see under
genitalia — male, 205
Urethral stricture, 113
Urethra opens under penis =
hypospadias, 30
Urethra, suturing of = urethror-
rhaphy, 57
Urethra, through the = trans-
urethral, 29
Urethra, to look in = urethroscopy,
53
Urethrorrhaphy, 57
Urethroscopy, 53
U.R.I., 227
Uria: see urine, 49
Urina, 71
Urinal, 71
Urinalysis: see under special
examinations, 207
Urinary and male genital systems,
diseases of, 112-113
Urinary bladder: see bladder,
urinary, under cystis, 70; also
see Ves. ur., 227
Urinary calculi, 113
Urinary system, anatomical parts,
109-110
Urinary tract: see urogenital
system, 109-118
Urinary tract stones = urinary
calculi, 113
Urinate, to: see ourein, 110; 156;
micturition, 170; voiding, 190
Urinating: see voiding, 190
Urine: see -uria, 49; albuminuria,
137; ouron, 109; 110; 136; 137;
140; 161; 172; 174; 178; 184;
urina, 71; also see abbr. Ur., 227
Urine, blood in = hematuria, 49;
161
Urine, chyle in = chyluria, 68

Urine collection in kidney pelvis =
hydronephrosis, 71
Urine incontinence, 163
Urine, much: see polyuria, 178
Urine output, uncontrolled: see
incontinence, 163
Urine, presence of indigo in =
indigouria, 35
Urine, protein in: see albuminuria,
137
Urine, purple-colored = porphyruria,
36
Urine, retention of: see under
genitourinary, 199
Urine, scanty = oliguria, 39; 174
Urine, suppression in kidney: see
anuria, 140
Urine, vessel for receiving = urinal,
71
Urine, voided drop by drop: see
strangury, 184
Urogenital, 217
Urogenital system, 70-72; 109-118
Urol., 227
Urologist, 23; 109; 110
Urology, 9; 14; 23; 227
Urticaria, 197; 239; 240; 241
U.S.P., 227
U.S.P.H.S., 227
Usual childhood diseases, 226
Uterine gestation, 72
Uterine hemorrhage independent of
menstruation = metrorrhagia, 48
Uterine hemorrhage with menstru-
ation: see menorrhagia, 117
Uterus, 4; 70; 114; 115; see also
under genitalia — female, 206; al-
so hystera (womb), 70; metra-, 4;
71; 180; 230
Uterus, curettage of, 51
Uterus, excessive bleeding between
menstruation = metrorrhagia, 117
Uterus, lining of = endometrium,
30; 115
Uterus, muscle structure of =
myometrium, 115
Uterus, neck of: see cervix, 71;
cervix uteri, 114
Uterus, outside covering of =
parametrium, 115
Uterus, positions of, 206
anteversion
prolapse
retroflexion
retroversion

Uterus, prolapse of: see under
descensus uteri, 233
Uterus, pus within the: see
pyometrium, 180
Uterus, suturing of = hysteror-
rhaphy, 57
Uterus, tumor (one type) of =
hysteromyoma, 70
Utricle, 131
Utterance: see phasis, 140
Uva., 106; 129
Uveal tract, 129
Uvula, 106; also see under mouth
and throat, 203

V

Va., 227
Vacca, 78; 189
Vaccine, 189
Vaccine, typhoid para A and B: see
T.A.B., 226
Vaccinia, 78
Vagare, 125
Vagina, 112; 115; also see colpos,
70; 230
Vagina and perineum, suturing of
= colpoperineorrhaphy, 57
Vaginal discharge: see under
genitourinary, 199
Vagina, suturing of = colpor-
rhaphy, 57
Vagus nerve, 125
Valve, mitral, 98
Valve, tricuspid, 98
Valvular disease: see leaking heart,
240
Valvular disease of heart, 227
Vand., 227
Van den Bergh, 227
Vanderbilt University Press, 249
V. and T., 227
var., 227
Vara, 92
Varicella = chickenpox, 81
Varicocele: see under genitalia —
male, 205
Varicose ulcers, 83
Varicose vein, obliteration of, 51
Varicose veins, 100; 189
Varicosities (varix): see under
breasts, 203; also under musculo-
skeletal system, 206

Variety, 227
Variola: see smallpox, 82; 245
Varix, 100; 189; see also varicose
veins, 100
Vas, 97; 112; 189
Vas-, 41
Vas deferens, 112
Vasospasm, 41; 131; 189
Vater, Abraham, 94
Vaultlike space: see fornix, 159
V.C., 227
V.D., 227
V.D.G., 227
V.D.H., 227
V.D.S., 227
Veil-like: see veli, 92
Vein, 98; see also phlebo, 67;
vena, 67; 98
Vein, dilatation of = phlebectasia,
27; varix, 189
Vein, inflammation of = phlebitis,
99
Vein, jugular, 98
Vein, opening of = phlebotomy, 67
Vein, saphenous, 98
Veins, enlarged and tortuous =
varicose veins, 100
Vein, small = venule, 67
Vein, suturing of = phleborrhaphy,
56
Veins, varicose, 100; 189
Veli, 92
Vena, 67; 98
Venereal, 199
Venereal disease, 227
Venereal disease, gonorrhea, 227
Venereal disease, syphilis, 227
Venereophobia, 237
Venous distention: see under neck,
203
Venter, 98; 190
Ventilare, 190
Ventilation, 190
Ventral, 190
Ventricle, 98; 190
Ventriculus, 190
Venule, 67
Verdin, 35
Verdohemin, 35
Vermiform, 190
Vermiform appendix: see appendix,
102
Vermifuge, 46

Vomiting, excessive, of pregnancy: see hyperemesis gravidarum, 242

Vomit with blood = hematemesis, 68

Von Recklinghausen's disease: see osteitis fibrosa cystica, 93

Von Roentgen, Wilhelm Konrad, 21

V.R., 227

Vulva, 115

Vulva and perineum, suturing of = episioperineorrhaphy, 57

Vulva, pruritus of, 118

V.W., 227

W

Wakefulness, abnormal: see egersis, 247

Walk about, able to: see ambulare, 138; 183; ambulant, 138

Walk, not able to: see abasia, 135

Wall: see paries, 78

Wander, to: see vagare, 125

Wart: see verruca, 190; 247

Waste, to cast out: see void, 190

Wasting: see tabes, 127

Wasting away: see emaciation, 155

Wasting palsy: see progressive muscular atrophy, 247

Water: see hydr-, 38; 162; aqua, 127; hydor, 152; 162; lympha, 168; see also aq., 211; H_2O, 218

Water ball: see cyst, 247

Water, common: see aqua communis, 211

Water, craving for = polydipsia, 134

Water cure: see hydrotherapy, 247

Water, distilled: see aqua distillata, 212

Water head: see hydrocephaly, 247

Water, loss of: see dehydration, 152

Water on knee: see hydrarthrosis, 247

Water, treatment by = hydrotherapy, 38

Wax: see cera, 147

Wax in ears: see cerumen, 147; 247; also see under ears, 201; 233

W.B.C. (w.b.c.), 227; see also under special examinations, 207

w-d, 227

Weakness: see asthenia, 141

Weakness, neurogenic: see under neuropsychiatric, 199

Weal: see wheal, 190; 248

Weariness: see kopos, 174

Weaver's bottom: see bursitis of gluteal bursa, 247

Weave, to: see plectere, 125

Weber's test: see A.C. and B.C., 210

Web-fingers: see syndactylism, 247

Weblike (of tissues): see hist-, 38; see also pannus, 176

Webster's New International Dictionary, 2; 250

Weight, 228

Well-being, sense of: see euphoria, 244

Well-developed, 227

Well-nourished, 227

Wen: see steatoma, 82; 248

West Publishing Co., 1; 249

Wetting bed: see enuresis, 156; 230

W.F., 227

Wheal, 190; 248

Wheezes, 248; see also wheezing under cardiorespiratory, 198

Whenever necessary, 223

While the pain lasts, 215

White: see alb-; albumin-; leuc-; leuk-, 34; also see leukos, 166

White blood cells: see leukocyte, 46; 227

White cells eating up red cells, 248

White female, 227

Whitehead: see steatoma, 82; 248

White leg: see milk leg, 241

White lines: see lineae albicantes, 167

White male, 227

White patchy areas: see under mouth and throat, 202

Whites: see leucorrhea, 233; 248

White swelling: see tuberculous abscess, 248

White, to be: see albicare, 167

Whitlow or felon: see paronychia, 248

Whooping cough: see pertussis, 34; 189; 248

Widening: see aneurysm, 138

Williams and Wilkins Co., 76; 249

Winchell, Walter, XI; 5; 240; 250

Windpipe: see trachea, 67; also see under bronchus, 95

Wind, puff of: see flatus; flatulence, 158

Winglike: see pterygoideus, 91
Wink, to = palpebrate, 74; 248
Witch's milk: see mastitis
  neonatorum, 248
With (together): see:
  co-, 29
  com-, 29
  con-, 29; 128; 151
  sym-, 29
  syn-, 29; 116; 185
  also see symbol (c̄), 213
Within: see:
  endo-, 7; 30; 101; 115
  ento-, 30
  intra-, 30
  intro-, 163
  intus-, 104
Without (lacking): see:
  a-, 31; 136; 140; 141; 142
  agenesis, 136
  an-, 31; 140
  e-, 155
  see also s̄., 225
W.M., 227
w-n, 227
Wolf: see lykos, 168
Woman: see gyn-, 38
Woman, study of diseases of =
  gynecology, 38
Womb: see:
  hystera, 70
  metra, 4; 71
  uterus, 4; 72; 115
Womb, dropped: see descensus
  uteri, 233
Word blindness: see alexia, 137
Words, inability to recall: see
  lethologica, 166
Words or phrases to name diseases
  common to anatomical systems,
  75-132
Words or phrases used to denote
  anatomical parts of each system,
  75-132
Words or phrases used to denote
  anatomical systems, 75-132
Word stems, medical, 61-74
Worm: see vermis, 102; 190; 248
Worm expeller = vermifuge, 46
Wormlike: see lumbricus, 90;
  vermiform, 190
Wound, a: see trauma, 188
Wounds, dirty, cleaning of =
  debridement, 56

Wrinkle: see rhytis, 248
Wrinkle, excision of: see
  rhytidectomy, 248
Wrist: see carpus, 65
Writer's cramps = chirospasm, 65;
  or see under cheirospasm, 248
Writing, a: see -gram, 46; -graphy,
  47
Wryneck = torticollis, 95
Wt., 228

X

X., 228
Xanth-, 35; 191
Xanthodont, 35
Xanthoma, 191
Xanthosis, 245
Xenophobia, 236
Xerasia, 238
Xeroderma, 191; 245
Xeros, 191
Xerosis, 191
Xiphoid, 191
Xiphoid process, 191
Xiphos, 191
X-ray: see radiology, 14; 21-22
X-ray dosage, unit of: see X., 228
X-ray of kidney pelvis and ureter =
  pyelogram, 71

Y

-y, 44
Yellow: see cirrh-, 35; lutein, 35;
  114; xanth-, 35; 191; jaune, 164
Yellow janders: see jaundice, 248
Yellow spot on retina, 228
Young in appearance: see agerasia,
  229
y.s., 228

Z

Zoon, 111
Zoophobia, 234
Zoster, 126; 191
Zygomatic arch, 88

♀ : see female, 228
♂ : see male, 228